Carb Cycling Diet

Table of Contents

Introduction

I want to thank you and congratulate you for downloading the book, *"Carb Cycling Diet"*

Carb cycling is truly a very interesting diet. When done the right way, you would not only enjoy the diet, but you would also achieve fast and sustainable results.

However, the key to unlock the potential benefits of carb cycling is doing it the right way. Ensure that you apply the principles you have learnt in this book and use it to develop a plan that would work for you.

The recipes in this book are easy to understand and prepare, so you don't have to worry if you are not a cooking-pro because the recipes have been given to you in a step-by-step manner. When you cook your own food, it is easier to track what you are eating and you don't need to worry if you are eating right and healthy. Each of the recipes are based on the basic foundation which includes the low-carb and high-carb variations.

The recipes are still customizable. You have a lot of endless possibilities in creating delicious and healthy meals.

Losing weight is not just about eating healthy foods but also eating the right portions. While there are a lot of applications that you can download to help you keep track of the amount of calories that you eat, it is still important that you know how portioning works.

Thanks again for downloading this book, I hope you enjoy it!

Chapter 1: History of carb cycling

Those who have been trying to lose excess pounds are probably familiar with the more popular diet fads, diet craze and diet menu plans. These diet plans' popularity stems from their promise of helping users to lose weight fast. These plans have different concepts and attacks.

Among the most recognizable are the low-carb diet plans that promise people that they will receive immediate positive results. However, some of those who tried these types of diet plans reported gaining the weight they lost right after reintroducing carbohydrates into their diets.

From popular trainer and transformation specialist, Chris Powell, comes carb cycling, a diet plan that alternates high-carb and low-carb days. How is it different from all the other weight loss plans before it?

There was a time in the 1970s and 1980s called the 'highcarb mania'. Most of the popular diets of that time encouraged the intake of large amounts of carbohydrates. However, this perception changed drastically in the 1990s and an exact opposite became popular. The diets of the 1990s, and later, concentrated on reducing the carbohydrate in the diet, giving rise to the 'lowcarb mania'. With that said, people are still unclear about how the carbs are used up in the human body. More precisely, the contribution of carb amounts to any weight loss program needs to be understood. Without any understatement, it can be said that your carb intake can be the game changer in your weight loss program and be responsible for weight loss.

On the other hand, it might just be the macronutrient that can destroy your plan completely. Today, the scenario has changed and there are a plethora of resources available for people to study and know what their bodies are going through, with and without a weight loss regime. Despite this availability of resources, people are still facing weight issues so much so that obesity is one of the most common problems faced by the world today.

This brings us to question as to why the scenario is deteriorating. After much contemplation, experts have stated that the reason behind the increasing problem of obesity is that none of the existing fitness systems understands the functioning of the human body. Most of the existing dietary approaches end up lowering the body's metabolism. As a result, the body loses all its energy and motivation to lose weight.

Franco Carlotto created carb cycle regiment in the 1990s, in his attempt to prepare for the Mr. World Fitness Title. In the process, he also helped millions of people around the world in maintaining a lean and healthy body. The main objective of this dietary approach was to help people achieve not just their long-term weight loss goals, but to reach both the short-term and long-term milestones in time. This technique has been developed from the analysis of how our ancestors ate and depleted their carb storage to maintain a healthy body. Although, the times have changed, the human body and the way it functions remains the same.

Therefore, the solution to weight loss issues also remains the same in the 21st century. We have to understand and manipulate our own carb storage system to get the weight loss results we expect. The carb cycle approach requires an individual to alternate high carb and low carb cycles on a daily basis, regulating the natural storage system of the body in such a way that the body doesn't store anything and burns more than what is expected on a daily and weekly basis. The low carb days deplete the body of its carbohydrates. However, the high carb days replenish the carb reserves. In this way, the body doesn't get exhausted of its energy and resources at any time. On a personal level, you don't have to give up on all your carbohydrate rich foods altogether. You just have to reduce there intake.

Chapter 2: What is carb cycling?

This has probably got you curious and wondering what carb cycling is all about. Carb cycling is simply an eating plan that lets you alternate between high carbs and low carbs on different days.

Your body makes use of different classes of food to perform its various functions. Protein for instance, is used for bodybuilding while carbohydrate supplies your body with the energy it needs to function. However, excess carbohydrate in the body is stored as fat therefore eating too much of carbohydrate without burning it through exercise or physical activity may increase the amount of fat in the body.

This is why some people choose to avoid carbohydrates altogether. However, completely avoiding carbohydrates would not do your body any good neither will it make you lose weight effectively. Although you may shed the pounds faster, there are a few downsides to that.

For one, you would be robbing your body of the essential nutrients and fiber that it needs. Also, low or no-carb diets are hardly sustainable. Therefore, it is almost impossible to achieve long-term weight loss on such diets.

Another downside of low-carb diets is that carbohydrates are actually replaced with other classes of foods like fats and proteins and this may lead to an increase in cholesterol levels thereby increasing risk of cardiovascular diseases.

There are so many other negative effects of low carb diets such as dizziness, fatigue, nausea, bad breath, and headache, which occur because of the body going into a state of ketosis.

Your body goes into a state of ketosis when you eat less than 20 grams of carbohydrates daily. Eating less than 20 grams of carbohydrates daily causes the body to switch from using carbohydrates as a source of energy to using stored fat in the body. This causes ketones to accumulate in the body and lead to the negative effects mentioned above.

On a carb cycling diet however, you do not have to cut down on carbs altogether; rather, you would control the way you consume your carbs. You would alternate your carbohydrate consumption in such a way that on some days, you eat foods that are very rich in carbohydrates while on some days, you go for foods with low carbohydrate content.

Eating this way helps to improve your metabolism so that your body begins to burn more calories. The healthy carbs, which you consume on this diet, would also help to control your blood sugar, reduce cravings, and improve your energy levels.

You do not feel weak or hungry as with other diets that have their principles based on starvation.

Carb Cycling Plans

There are four different carb cycling plans, which you should know about. They include:

Easy Carb Cycle

As a beginner, you should start with the Easy Carb Cycle. The Easy Carb Cycle is a very effective plan for people who find it hard to cut out on certain foods.

Are you the type who loves pizza so much that the thought of not having it in a week makes you dread any form of diet at all? Then the Easy Carb Cycle is for you.

This carb-cycling plan allows you to alternate between high carb and low carb days and on your high carb days; you are allowed to enjoy your favorite foods or snacks that you crave as long as you don't have them at dinner.

So yes, you can have cakes, chips, ice cream, or anything you want and still lose weight. The only rule is that you can only have these things as a REWARD MEAL on your HIGH-CARB DAYS.

Sounds easy, right? It's actually easy.

Another rule is that you have to spread your meals throughout the day. Instead of eating three heavy meals a day, you should have at least five small meals throughout the day. And this applies to both high-carb and low carb days. This further helps to boost your metabolism and helps you burn more calories.

So on an easy carb cycle, this is what your eating plan would look like:

Sunday
Reward meal
High carb day

Monday
Low carb day

Tuesday
Reward meal
High carb day

Wednesday
Low carb day

Thursday

Reward meal

High carb day

Friday

Low carb day

Saturday

Reward meal

High Carb day

Remember, if you are craving anything, anything at all, you don't have to deprive yourself; all you need to do is to move it up to your high carb day or eat it as your reward meal.

You can move up to another carb cycling plan or you can stay with this plan throughout your diet; the decision is entirely yours to make.

Classic Carb Cycle

The classic carb cycle is a step higher than the easy carb cycle but is just as easy and effective for weight loss as the easy carb cycle.

On the classic carb cycle, you are allowed one whole day to satisfy all your cravings. This day serves as your reward day. So instead of having a reward meal every other day as with the easy carb cycle, you would have one full day to satisfy all your cravings.

The good thing is that you would still be able to alternate between the high and the low carb days.

This is what your eating plan on a classic carb cycle would look like:

Sunday

Reward day

Monday

Low carb day

Tuesday

High carb day

Wednesday

Low carb day

Thursday

High carb day

Friday

Low carb day

Saturday

High carb day

On this cycle, you are able to lose weight quickly and constantly. You may also choose to remain on this cycle throughout your weight loss journey or move up to another carb-cycling plan.

Turbo Cycle

The Turbo cycle helps you lose weight faster than all the other carb cycles. Instead of alternating high carb days with low carb days as you do on other plans, on the turbo cycle, you would have to put in two low carb days for every high carb day. So, in a week you get four low carb days, two high carb days and one reward day.

This type of eating plan helps you burn fat consistently for two days before re-stoking on your high carb day.

The turbo cycle is also very powerful in the sense that you do not have to restrict your calories. Women can have at least 1,200 calories a day while men can have at least 1,500 calories daily.

This is what your eating plan on a turbo cycle would look like:

Sunday

Reward day

Monday

Low carb day

Tuesday

Low carb day

Wednesday

High carb day

Thursday

Low carb day

Friday

Low carb day

Saturday

High carb day

The turbo cycle is a powerful weight loss accelerator and you may decide to stay on this plan throughout your weight loss journey or move on to another cycle.

The Fit Cycle

The fourth carb-cycling plan is the fit cycle. This is the best carb-cycling plan for people who are highly active physically such as athletes, body builders, and trainers.

The fit cycle plan helps you eliminate fat while supplying your body with the fuel, which it needs to perform. There are only two low carb days a week in this cycle.

On the extra high carb days, your body is able to absorb more glycogen, which serves as energy for high performance. This is alternated by the low carb days when the body's supply of glycogen has been depleted and the muscles have developed insulin-sensitivity thereby allowing it to soak up more carbs and burn extra calories on the high carb and reward days.

The fit cycle eating plan would look like this:

Sunday
Reward day

Monday
High carb day

Tuesday
High carb day

Wednesday
Low carb day

Thursday
High carb day

Friday
High carb day

Saturday
Low carb day

The fit cycle allows you to lose weight and burn fat without compromising on your physical performance. You would still get all the energy you need to achieve your athletic goals while losing weight rapidly.

Chapter 3: Why carb cycle?

Carb cycling helps you structure your carb consumption in such a way that you do not eat too little so that it begins to slow down your metabolism and you do not eat too much either.

Here are a few reasons why carb cycling is the best diet for you or anyone who is really serious about losing weight the healthy way;

Carb Cycling Promotes Fat Burning

On a carb cycling diet, you would not just lose water weight as with most traditional diets; you would actually lose fat.

Carb cycling enables your body to burn fat as fuel as opposed to just burning carbohydrates and muscle tissues.

Carb Cycling Helps You Build Lean Muscles

Carb cycling also helps you to get leaner while building muscles. This is because carb cycling helps to make your body better at controlling insulin so that more glucose is stored in the muscles instead of fat cells.

Carb Cycling Increases Receptiveness to Insulin

The high carb days helps to stimulate insulin response so that nutrients are moved to your muscle cells causing them to grow while the low carb days makes your body much more responsive to insulin.

Carb Cycling Helps You Reduce Consumption of Bad Carbs

All carbs are not created equal. There are the good and healthy carbs and there are the not-so healthy ones. The unhealthy carbs increase blood glucose levels and make you hungry and crave unhealthy foods like candy, fries, and other snacks. Carb cycling helps you consume less of these unhealthy carbs and more of healthy carbs like whole grains, oats, fruits, legumes, and whole oats.

Carb Cycling is Easy

Carb cycling is not like any of the diets that leave you starving, weak, and unable to concentrate. You actually get to eat the foods you love while losing weight.

You can actually go out with your friends, go out on dinner dates, and still enjoy regular meals while you are on the diet. What can be better than this?

How to determine if Carb Cycling is Safe for You

There's sad news here. Carb cycling works and is one of the easiest and most effective diet plans for weight loss currently.

But sadly, carb cycling is not for everyone. Carb cycling is only good for people who want to use it as a short-term approach to weight loss.

Most nutritionists and health experts advice that carb cycling should only be done for a short period of at most four months.

Doing the carb recycling diet for longer than this may affect the body negatively.

Participating in the carb cycling diet program can help you prevent sudden dips in your metabolic rate.

This diet program can help you to prevent imbalances in your digestive system. In the process, you keep yourself from feeling bloated, regardless of the cycle of the diet program that you are currently in.

This diet program helps you to decrease the average amount of carbohydrates that you consume within a certain period of time.

Your body will not have to deal with excessive glycogen levels that will most likely not be utilized for the rest of the day. This will give your liver and your pancreas some much-needed rest. Because of this, you can prevent medical conditions such as diabetes mellitus. Some studies have also shown that decreased exposure to high glycogen levels helps to prevent cardiovascular system disorders from bring harmful.

As for leptin production, you can expect to have more as you go along with carb cycling.

Leptin is a substance that can help to regulate your hunger. Therefore, leptin can help you have decreased incidences of food cravings. In the process, you can expect your metabolism to significantly increase. This can lead to better weight management overall and the effective shedding of fat tissue.

Because of food item regulation and regular exercise, you can expect a steady boost in biochemicals, which can assist you in breaking down the fat tissue stored in your body.

While participating in this diet program, you can expect increased levels of testosterone and HGH in your body. This can help you to break down fat molecules by improving the growth rates of major muscle groups. These can also help you increase your metabolic rate for an even more effective fat breakdown process.

Helps to promote the entire process of fat loss.

Aside from fat breakdown evident through food amount and type regulation, you must make changes in your physical activity levels. Specifically, you must increase the intensity of the exercises that you perform in order to help you to develop your muscle groups. The difficulties of the workout routines that you need to perform are directly proportional to the fat breakdown potentials through carbohydrate and nutrient consumption.

In relation to the previous point, carb cycling can help you to prevent gaining more fat than allowed.

More protein means more building blocks for your major muscle groups. This can translate to larger muscle masses overall. Because your muscles will be larger, they will consume more energy sources in order to keep them going. Fat tissue is a major source of energy for these muscles. As you work out more, and consume protein, you will lose more adipose tissue. In the process, you will develop a leaner body mass.

The longer you adhere to the diet program; you can expect your glycogen restoration levels to have improvements.

Because your diet program helps with significant improvements for your major muscle groups, you can expect that these muscle groups will also use up more glycogen. This is what happens when you participate in this diet program. As your muscles get bigger, the amount of dormant energy reserves decrease. When this happens, excessive adipose tissue is eventually obliterated.

As soon as you get used to carb cycling, it will be easier for you to keep doing exercises with a high intensity.

As much as the diet program helps to increase the amount of fat that your body uses up, it is much easier for your body to pace the energy usage. In other words, there is a better distribution of energy sources when you perform physical activity. This especially holds true when you are required to perform relatively difficult exercise routines for a prolonged period of time.

Because of the promising benefit of fat breakdown, this diet program can help you to develop and maintain a lean body form.

After you have noticed the significant improvements for your body, you will notice that there are major improvements on the functionalities of your muscles overall. This can be more convenient because you can easily perform the tasks that you must do. The good news is that you get to perform these tasks even better than they were performed before.

This diet program can keep your muscles and bones from deteriorating.

As your muscles begin to develop, you will have a better chance of using them for most of your tasks. When this happens, there is a good chance of developing them by virtue of "constant pressure". Moreover, your body has a good chance of gaining the right nutrients which can help to prevent further bone and muscle deterioration.

Carb cycling can help in muscle growth and development.

Due to the fact that there is a fixed amount of minimum protein consumption that you must take for every meal, your body has a virtually unlimited supply of amino acids. Amino acids are substances that your body can use for muscle reinforcement and repair. Coupled with the right exercise, you can enjoy larger and leaner muscle mass within four to six weeks.

Unlike other diet programs out there, this program can help you to prevent adaptation over time.

Preventing adaptation over time is extremely helpful because it can help you to prevent any weight regain. Because of the unpredictability in diet and workout modifications, there comes a time in which your body will guess on what comes next.

This diet program can prevent plateaus from occurring.

Since this diet program is somewhat unpredictable, you are able to dodge the possibility of exponentially decreasing benefits and negative health impacts.

You will not experience food deprivation because of the balanced meal plans suggested.

Although it seems like food deprivation is stressed because of food choice restrictions described in the book, your body will not feel deprived because it receives a complete set of nutrients for each day. Therefore, your body will not seek more food items in the long run.

In relation to the previous point, you will have a prolonged satiety period.

Satiety takes place because most of the recommended food items included in the diet have delayed processing capacities in the stomach. This means that these specific food items will induce a longer digestion time for your body. The stomach will send a signal to the brain that it is still full after some time. The brain will then send impulses that will tell your stomach to keep on processing the food items and absorbing the nutrients from these food items.

Food cravings will never be an issue once you take part in this diet program.

On this diet, you are exposed to decreased levels of refined carbohydrates. Refined carbs are included in those food groups in which your digestive system can easily break down. More food items will eventually lead to glycogen pile up. Fortunately, you do not have to suffer this fate if you participate in the diet program because the meal plans satisfy you and with this, you have less chance of gaining weight.

Chapter 4: How carb cycling works

Carb cycling, also known as carbohydrate cycling, is a weight management technique that requires certain meal plans to be incorporated with regulated types of food groups in them. Usually, the food items included in the meal plans are monitored for carbohydrate content. As the name of the diet program implies, carbohydrate-laden food items are important to monitor because they determine the type of food item that will be eaten for each meal on any given day.

There are different aspects to the carbohydrate cycle that you should understand.

You should keep in mind that there are six meals that you have to consume each day. Each of the meals eaten should have regular intervals between each other. This will help to ensure that you develop a regular and highly functional metabolic rate for your digestive system.

During a high carb-laden day, you are allowed to consume as many carbohydrates as you want, but only for certain meals within the day.

Out of the six meals that you will eat on that day, you may consume as many carbs as you desire for four of the meals. You may eat carbs as soon as you have consumed the recommended amount of fats and proteins.

Aside from your unlimited carbohydrate consumption, you must eat a piece of fruit with 50 to 100 calories before you consume any carbs.

The fruit you consume contains fructose that will help your body to produce more energy. The body can produce more energy by virtue of glycogen storage inside your liver. Even if fructose is a form of sugar, this cannot affect the fat production in your body because the consumption of 50 to 100 calories is not enough to elicit an effect in your body. Instead, the fructose value that you consume can help promote prolonged satiety for your digestive system. Thus, you will have a decreased need to eat additional meals in between the predetermined six meals on this specific day. And, this will prevent you from overeating.

The Low- carbs day may be considered as the most complicated among the three phases of this diet program due to certain macronutrient goals that you must fulfill.

For this specific carb cycling day, you must consume carbohydrates for only three out of the six meals that you eat. Before you consume any carbohydrates, you need to include the prescribed amount of protein and fat in your diet. Moreover, you must consume a small fruit with 50 to 100 calories in it beforehand.

The recommended amount of carbohydrates is set at one gram of carbs for every one pound of weight in your body each day. After computing for the total value of carbs that you must consume each day, you would then divide this value by three. This is the amount of carbs that you are allowed to eat for three out of the six meals during your low carbs day. You should note that the amount of carbs that you need to consume for each meal should be equally distributed in order to ensure consistency in your metabolic rate.

A no-carbs day is considered the easiest, but most important, among the phases of carb cycling.

The no-carbs day is regarded as the most controversial part of the carbs cycling diet program. As the term suggests, you are not allowed to eat any food items with carbs for the six meals that you will have for that day. But, you still need to consume the minimum amount of fat and protein for all your meals to prevent delaying your muscle development process. Apart from these instructions, you may consume as much protein as you want for your meals on this day.

Initially, you may find it difficult to get through this day. One way to keep on track is to motivate yourself by thinking about the high carbs day that lies only a few days ahead.

There are numerous factors which can determine if you will emerge successful while engaging in the carbs cycling diet program.

You are able to control some of these factors of the diet program. But, you cannot manipulate the other factors of this diet because they are fixed and based on the specific genetic aspects of your body.

If you want to build a solid foundation in order to ensure success for your diet program, setting certain diet related goals can help you do this.

Your goals will determine the success rate that you will attain at the end of the diet program, once you complete the program. Experts recommend that you adhere to a set time, as well as realistic, objective, specific, and concrete goals. Composing your goals in this manner will help you to stay motivated. These goals will help you to assess your progress during the time you are on the diet.

Before you start off with the actual diet program, you should set your long term and short term goals. In the process of goal setting, you should already know what you want to attain after the program. In the long run, this will tell you how much satisfaction you will attain after reaching your goals.

Body builds are uncontrollable variables that can somehow determine your success rate in the carb cycling diet program.

Different body types have different reactions to certain diet programs that are introduced. Therefore, you must have your body type assessed in order to determine how you use the program to create significant and positive results for your body.

- Ectomorphic is known as the thin body type. People with this body type have a small and rather delicate body frame and bone structure. Experts do not usually recommend this diet program for people with ectomorphic body types because they already have high metabolic rates used to get rid of the adipose tissues in their body.

- Mesomorphic is known as the lean body type. People with this body type have naturally athletic physiques. Given this fact, mesomorphs usually manifest with large muscle groups and sturdy bone structures.

- Endomorphic is the soft and solid body type. Compared to the two previous body types presented, the endomorphic body type tends to have the largest proportions of fat. People with this body type are the most sensitive to carbohydrates. This implies that they should consume fewer carbohydrates because they tend to gain more fats compared to the mesomorphs and the ectomorphs. Given these premises, endomorphs have the most weight management benefits if they maximize the intricacies of the program.

Your lifestyle can tell you how successful you will be on this diet program even before you start.

For most diet programs out there, you must also incorporate various workout routines and physical activities into your daily schedule. This activity is important because it will set your major muscle groups to work. As soon as they are set to work, you initiate the processes of fat breakdown and muscle buildup. You must do these things for the rest of your life.

Support systems can mean a lot, especially when you are going through difficult phases of your carb cycle.

Working with a support system can make you accountable for everything that you are about to do which is related to your diet program. The right support system reminds you to fulfill your goals and plans. They can also affirm and encourage you when you are successful. If you are doing something that can benefit you in the long run, they will let you know. Some support systems can even assist you in creating diet and exercise alternatives.

Like other diet programs out there, the carb cycling diet includes different goals for each phase that you go through while in the cycle.

The main goal of this diet program is to help you lose those unwanted pounds. In the process, carb cycling should help you to develop lean muscle mass instead of wasting muscle mass. As soon as you see that you are getting rid of fats while toning up your body, you will eventually get motivated to continue the program.

Monitoring your progress as you go along the diet program can help you to further boost your motivation levels. To help you monitor your achievements while participating in the program, you have to weigh yourself and take measurements regularly, such as hip to waist ratio and waistline measurements. You must obtain baseline measurements for these aspects as these will serve as the base of comparisons for your next measurements. Afterward, you will need to take measurements every six to eight weeks that you are on the diet. On average, each cycle of this diet program lasts for three to four days.

Because workouts are considered a part of any type of effective diet program, you should make specific considerations when working out while you are involved in the carb cycling diet program.

Right after performing all your workout routines, you will have to consume 30 to 50 grams worth of protein. This will help to reinforce the process of muscle development and assist you in muscle repair. If you are on a low carbs or high carbs day, during the day of the workout, you have to follow up your protein intake with some carbohydrates. If you want to yield better results, you have to consume food items such as whey protein and oatmeal.

Chapter 5: How much to eat and of what?

What you can Include in Your Diet

Aside from the recipes above, you will have examples of carb-cycling foods that you are allowed to have:

Protein:
Beef
- Cube steak – 2.5 oz
- Low sodium roast beef - 3 oz
- Extra lean sirloin steak – 2 oz
- Lean flank steak – 2.5 oz
- Venison – 2 oz

Dairy
- Cottage cheese ½ cup
- Egg whites – 4 whites
- Egg substitutes – 1 cup
- Plain Greek yogurt -3/4 cup

Lean Ground Meats
- Extra lean ground beef – 2 oz
- Ground chicken breast – 4 oz
- Ground turkey – 3 oz

Poultry
- Duck breast – 2 oz
- Skinless chicken thigh – 3 oz
- Skinless chicken breast – 3.5 oz

Powdered
- Whey, soy, hemp, rice – 1 scoop

Fish
- Salmon fillet – 2 oz
- Sardines – 52 g (4 sardines)
- Canned tuna – 3 oz
- Tuna fillet – 3 oz
- White fish – 2.5 oz

Shellfish
- Raw clams – 5 oz
- Shrimp/lobster – 4 oz

Vegetable Protein
- Tempeh – 2 oz
- Tofu – 4 oz

White Meat
- Pork tenderloin – 2.5 oz

Carbohydrates:
Bread
- Corn tortillas – 1 ½ servings
- Bread – 1 slice
- English muffin – ½ piece

Cereal
- Low-fat granola – ½ cup

- Old-fashioned oatmeal (cooked) – ¾ cup

Grains
- Buckwheat, Bran, Barley, Brown Rice – ½ cup
- Oats (steel-cut, cooked) – 2/3 cup
- Popcorn (no oil) – 3 cups
- Quinoa – ½ cup
- Wild rice – ½ cup

Legumes
- Beans – ½ cup
- Lentils – ½ cup
- Soybeans – ¼ cup
- Soy nuts - 3 tbsp

Pasta
- Brown rice pasta – ½ cup
- Couscous – ½ cup
- Whole grain – ½ cup

Root Vegetables
- Carrots – 2 cups
- Potatoes – ¾ cup
- Beets – 1 ½ cups
- Yams and sweet potatoes – 2/3 cup

Starchy Vegetables
- Peas – 1 cup
- Corn - 2/3 cup

Fruits:
Fresh
- Apricots – 6 pieces
- Banana – 1 piece

- Apples – 1 ½
- Berries, like blueberries, cherries, and strawberries – 1 ½ cups
- Grapes – 1 ½ cups
- Oranges – 1 piece
- Melons – 1 ½ cups
- Mangoes – 1 cup
- Lemons and limes – 5 pieces
- Papayas – 2 cups
- Plums – 3 ½ pieces
- Pineapple – ½ cup
- Peaches – 2 large pieces
- Pears – 1 piece
- Grapefruit – 1 piece
- Kiwi – 4 pieces

Vegetables:
- Asparagus – 3 ½ cups
- Artichokes – 2 pieces, medium-sized
- Broccoli – 4 cups
- Brussels sprouts – 2 ½ cups
- Bok Choy – 1 head
- Cabbage – 4 cups
- Chard – 10 leaves
- Celery – 5 cups
- Cauliflower – 4 cups
- Collard greens – 10 cups
- Eggplant – 5 cups
- Garlic – 20 cloves
- Fennel – 4 cups
- Green beans – 75 pieces
- Kale – 3 cups
- Mushrooms – 20 large pieces
- Leeks – 2 pieces
- Okra – 2 pieces medium-sized

- Radish – 5 cups
- Scallions – 10 cups
- Snow peas – 70 pods
- Parsley – 4 cups
- Spinach – 10 cups
- Tomatoes – 6 ½ pieces, medium-sized
- Turnips – 2 large pieces
- Zucchini – 2 large pieces

Fats:
Dairy:
- Cream cheese – 2 tbsp
- Egg yolk – 2
- Whip cream – 2 tbsp
- Mozzarella – 1 oz
- Parmesan – 1 oz
- Romano – 1 oz

Nuts and Seeds:
- Almonds – 1 ½ tbsp
- Peanut butter – 1 tbsp
- Pecans – 1 ½ tbsp
- Sesame seeds – 2 tbsp
- Sunflower seeds – 1 ½ tbsp

Beverages:
- Black coffee – unlimited
- Unsweetened soy milk – 1 ¼ cup
- Tea (herbal, green) – unlimited
- Water – unlimited
- Tomato juice – 2 ½ cups

Now that you have been given easy to follow and prepare carb cycling food recipes, you don't have any excuse to lose weight. Don't worry if you cannot cook all the time because of work and household chores, you can bulk-prepare your foods and store in the fridge. You can easily reheat and eat!

It is important to know some of the food items that you can incorporate in your meal plans. Some of these particular food items are included in this section.

Despite the fact that it contains fat, avocados can bring you a lot of diet related benefits.

Avocados are in fiber that which helps to flush out the harmful toxins inside your body. They also contain foliate, potassium, and mono-saturated fats.

Brown rice may be a bit expensive at the store, but it can help you reap many weight loss benefits in the long run.

Brown rice is rich in dietary fiber and manganese. Manganese is considered a catalyst for carbohydrate and proteins. And, it works well with your nervous system.

Garlic is a wonder food and drug that even ancient people used.

You may incorporate garlic in your dishes if you cannot afford to eat it by itself. You may also take garlic capsules to enjoy garlic's benefits without consuming in the natural form.

Chicken serves as one of the most versatile food items that you can add into your diet.

Chicken contains nutrients such as vitamin B3, vitamin B6, selenium, and phosphorus. Chicken is also rich in protein and dietary fiber.

Milk is a complete food that can help with numerous health-related issues.

Milk can contribute to a stronger immune system, increased bone strength, and smoother skin, to name only a few benefits. Milk can also help people who are dealing with chronic illnesses.

Chapter 6: Forbidden Foods on the Carb Cycling Diet

Although these foods are forbidden, you can have them on your cheat/reward days;

- Refined or processed carbohydrates
- Brown sugar
- Corn syrup
- Raw sugar
- Ice cream
- Chocolates
- Candy
- Soda
- Refined/white flour
- Cake
- Cookies
- Pastries
- Donuts
- Crackers
- White bread
- White rice
- Chips
- Fried meals
- Hydrogenated oils
- Alcoholic beverages like wine and beer.
- Foods high in sodium
- Artificial sweeteners like saccharin, aspartame, and sucralose.

Chapter 7: Breakfast Recipes:

Superfoods Smoothie

Yield: Servings 3 | Serving Size: 1 Glass | Calories: 131 | Total Fat: 1 g | Saturated Fat: 0 g | Trans Fat: 0 g | Cholesterol: 2 mg | Sodium: 287 mg | Carbohydrates: 26 g | Dietary Fiber: 4 g | Sugars: 13 g | Protein: 7 g | SmartPoints: 5 |

INGREDIENTS

1 cup baby spinach loosely packed (organic)
1 sm frozen banana, slice before freezing
1 cup frozen berries, unsweetened (blueberries were used in the photo)
Fresh ginger root (1/2? slice)
1/2 cup Kefir or Greek Yogurt, plain, low-fat
1 cup chilled green tea (unsweetened)…home brewed is best.
1/2 cup pure pomegranate juice
1 cup crushed ice

DIRECTIONS

Toss all ingredients in the blender and blend until smooth. The blender will be filled to the top with loads of super foods, so be sure the lid is on securely before blending. It will take a minute or so for all the ingredients to blend completely.

For a thinner smoothie, add more green tea.

Enjoy and reap the benefits!!!

Yogurt and fresh fruit

Candied Maple Sweet Potatoes

Yields: 8 servings | Serving Size: ½ cup | Calories: 215 | Total Fat: 9 g | Saturated Fat: 1 g | Trans Fat: 0 g | Cholesterol: 0 mg | Sodium: 129 mg | Carbohydrates: 3g | Dietary Fiber: 4 g | Sugars: 9 g | Protein: 2 g | SmartPoints:8

INGREDIENTS

4 to 6 sweet potatoes, well-scrubbed or peeled and cut into 1/2 inch cubes

1/4 cup extra-virgin olive oil

1/4 cup pure maple syrup

2 teaspoons ground cinnamon

1 cup plumped raisins or dried cranberries

1 orange, juiced and zested*

1/4 teaspoon salt and freshly ground black pepper

DIRECTIONS

Preheat oven to 375 degrees F.

For the Candied Maple Sweet Potatoes:

Plump the raisins or dried cranberries by placing them in a bowl of hot water and allowing them to stand for 15 to 20 minutes, until softened.

Meanwhile, peel the orange into wide strips with a vegetable peeler. Halve the orange and squeeze the juice into the bottom of a large bowl.

Place the sweet potatoes and raisins (or dried cranberries) into the bowl, and toss with olive oil, orange peels, cinnamon, maple syrup, and salt and pepper.

Place the sweet potatoes in a single layer on a rimmed nonstick baking sheet, pouring any remaining liquid in the bowl evenly over the sweet potatoes. Bake for 20 to 25 minutes until cooked through and golden crisp on the outside.

Strawberry Banana Smoothie

Servings: 2 | Serving Size: 1/2 of the entire recipe | Calories: 250 | Total Fat: 5 g | Saturated Fats: 0 g | Trans Fats: 0 g | Cholesterol: 13 mg | Sodium: 28 mg | Carbohydrates: 41 g | Dietary fiber: 5.5 g | Sugars: 21 g | Protein: 13 g | SmartPoints: 9 |

INGREDIENTS

1 large frozen banana (slice into 1? pieces before freezing)
6 large frozen strawberries (unsweetened)
1/2 slice fresh ginger root (optional)
1 cup skim milk (almond or milk alternative**)
½ cup Greek Yogurt, plain fat free
1/4 cup wheat germ

DIRECTIONS

Place all the ingredients in a blender and blend until creamy…just like a milkshake. Add a straw and enjoy!

Breakfast Yogurt Parfait To Go

Servings: 3 | Serving Size: 1 cup | Calories: 184 | Total Fat: 8 g | Saturated Fats: 4 g | Trans Fats: 0 g | Cholesterol: 0 mg | Sodium: 35 mg | Carbohydrates: 23 g | Dietary Fiber: 4 g | Sugars: 1 g | Protein: 6 g | SmartPoints: 6 |

INGREDIENTS

1 cup grapes or mixed berries

1/2 banana, chopped

1/4 cup unsweetened shredded coconut

1/2 cup granola

1/2 cup nonfat or lowfat Greek-style yogurt

DIRECTIONS

Place a layer of berries or grapes on the bottom of the jar, add a layer of yogurt, a layer of granola, a layer of fruit, another layer of yogurt and a layer of the shredded coconut. Cap the jar, and off you go!

Individual Egg & Spinach Bowls

Yields: 4 servings | Serving Size: 1 bowl | Calories: 84 | Total Fat: 2 g | Saturated Fat: 1 g | Trans Fat: 0 g | Cholesterol: 57 | Carbohydrates: 6 g | Sodium: 335 mg | Dietary Fiber: 1 g | Sugars: 2 g | Protein: 11 g | SmartPoints: 2 |

INGREDIENTS

8 large egg whites, (recommend free-range)

1 whole egg

1 cup baby spinach, torn or chopped into small pieces

1/2 cup diced tomatoes

1/4 cup feta cheese, fat-free

1/2 teaspoon black pepper

Kosher or sea salt to taste

DIRECTIONS

Preheat oven to 350 degrees.

Whisk together all ingredients in a medium mixing bowl. Lightly mist 4 (1/2 cup) ramekins with nonstick cooking spray and evenly divide egg mixture into bowls.

Place ramekins on a cookie sheet and bake 20 minutes or until eggs puff and are almost set in the center. Serve hot.

Avocado Breakfast Pizzas served on low calorie tortilla

Yields: 2 Breakfast Pizzas | Serving Size: 1 Breakfast Pizza | Calories: 299 | Total Fat: 24 g | Saturated Fat: 4 g | Trans Fat: 0 g | Cholesterol: 186 mg | Sodium: 84 mg | Carbohydrates: 14 g | Dietary Fiber: 7 g | Sugars: 1 g | Protein: 9 g | SmartPoints: 9 |

INGREDIENTS

2 whole grain tortillas (6 inch diameter)
2 eggs
2 tsp olive oil
1 avocado, peeled and seeded
1 tsp lemon juice
salt and pepper, to taste

DIRECTIONS

First, warm tortillas in the microwave for approximately 30 seconds. Set aside.

In a small bowl, combine the avocado and lemon juice. Mix well until the mixture has a smooth consistency. Season with salt and pepper to taste.

Spread avocado mixture in an even layer on both tortillas. Set aside.

Heat a skillet greased with the olive oil at medium heat until just hot enough to sizzle a drop of water.

Break eggs and gently add to the skillet. Immediately reduce heat to low.

Cook slowly until whites are completely set and yolks begin to thicken but are not hard.

Place warm eggs on top of the tortillas and season with salt and pepper as desired.

Smoked haddock fillet with 2 poached eggs and asparagus.

INGREDIENTS

6 Asparagus Spears
Smoked Undyed Haddock Fillet (1-2 depending on your serving)
Bisto Chicken Stock Melt
2 Free Range Medium eggs
1 x Yellow Pecorino Pepper
Lemon Juice
A handful of fresh Dill
Fresh Coriander to garnish
1 Calorie Olive Oil Fry Light
Salt and Black Pepper

DIRECTIONS

1. Line a baking tray with foil (saves you washing up and stops the fish sticking to the tray)

    Put your fish skin down onto the tray.

    Lightly drizzle some lemon juice over the fish (Fresh or bottled is fine)

2. Next dust your fish with salt (I prefer Reduced Sodium Salt) and

cracked black pepper. This will stick to the lemon juice you have just drizzled.

3. Then cut your chives and dill quite roughly on a board and place over your fish to cover it. Put the tray into an oven on the top shelf for 25 minutes at gas mark 5.

4. Get your Asparagus ready on a chopping board. Purple Asparagus like this one will turn a lovely green when I show you a great method to cook it.

   Cut off the ends of the Asparagus. They are fine in soup but too woody for this dish.

   Cut your Asparagus into two.

5. Spray a non-stick griddle pan with Fry Light 1 Calorie Spray

6. Heat the pan and grill your Asparagus for 3 minutes. Then add a Bisto Chicken Stick Melt to the pan and add enough boiling water to cover the Asparagus. (About 1 cm deep will be fine). The water will bubble up. Take a spoon and stir in the stock melt.

   Turn the heat down to simmer lightly, turning the Asparagus over gently whilst cooking. The Asparagus will soak up all this juice and make them lovely and bright.

   This will only take 15 mins

7. Use a perfect poach egg kit to get perfect poached eggs. Wait until you have ten minutes left on your fish and your Asparagus are nearly done as it so quick.

   Then pop your egg into the kit Spray the inserts with Fry Light Olive Oil Spray.

   Then crack your eggs into the inserts. Turn the heat down on your saucepan hob to simmer and quickly put the poacher kit lid on top.

The great thing about this kit is you can see through the lid and keep an eye on your poached eggs. Your eggs will take exactly four mins so you can get your fish and Asparagus ready.

8. After 25 mins your fish will be ready. You can take it out to get to ready while your eggs are cooking. You will see the lemon juice has created a lovely golden juice and the dill will be slightly charred which gives it a great taste.

9. Then when you have your Haddock and Asparagus laid up ready on your plate then take the lid off the egg saucepan and turn off all heat, then pop the ege down on your plate.

10. Its fun to slightly cut the poached egg so that the yolk oozes out over the meal. Garnish with Coriander which will complement the smoky Haddock.

Enjoy and reap the benefits!!!

Scrambled eggs and lean bacon rashers.

INGREDIENTS

4 large beefsteak tomatoes
sea salt and freshly ground black pepper
1-2 tsp Demerara Sugar
2-3 rashers lean streaky bacon, per person
Scrambled Eggs (Per person)
2 eggs
2 Tbsp milk or cream
1 Tbsp chopped herbs, parsley, dill, chervil and or chives
salt and freshly ground black pepper

DIRECTION

Preheat oven to 200°C. Spray a roasting dish or ovenproof lasagne dish with non-stick baking spray. Slice tomatoes in half and sit cut side up in the tray. Sprinkle with sea salt & freshly ground black pepper and a pinch of demerara sugar.

Cook for 20 to 25 minutes. The sugar will have melted and caramelised on top but the tomatoes will still keep their shape. Bacon cooks really crispy in the oven and takes the same time as the tomatoes, so pop them in together while you prepare the scrambled eggs.

Roll rashers of lean streaky bacon into bundles and cook in a roasting dish or oven tray with a slightly raised edge. Drain on absorbent paper.

For the scrambled eggs, heat a large non-stick frypan over medium heat. Add a small teaspoon sized knob of butter if desired. Whisk eggs, milk, herbs and salt & freshly ground black pepper together. Pour into the heated pan and swirl around. Turn heat down to low and using a silicon spatula, stir eggs gently to cook. Serve while still quite soft and runny as they continue to cook when removed from the heat source.

If desired, serve on slices of wholemeal toast.

Oats

50g oats with 200ml skimmed milk. Serve with raspberries and honey. Stir in ½ scoop of whey protein at the end

Cheese Ham omelette

INGREDIENTS

2 eggs

2 Tbsp. fat-free milk

4 slices OSCAR MAYER Deli Fresh Smoked Ham, chopped

1 tsp. thinly sliced green onions

dash pepper

1/4 cup KRAFT 2% Milk Shredded Cheddar Cheese

DIRECTIONS

Whisk eggs and milk in small bowl until blended. Stir in ham, onions and pepper.

Pour into 8-inch nonstick skillet; cover. Cook on medium heat 6 min. or until egg mixture is set but top is still moist.

Sprinkle cheese onto half the omelet; fold in half. Remove from heat; let stand, covered, 1 min. Cut in half

Omelet Egg whites 3
INGREDIENTS
1 tablespoon Unsalted Butter
1/4 cup finely chopped red and/or green bell peppers
1 tablespoon finely chopped onion
1/2 cup pasteurized liquid egg whites
2 ounces (1/4 cup) Cheddar Cheese, shredded

DIRECTIONS
1. Melt butter in 8-inch skillet until sizzling; add bell peppers and onions. Cook over medium heat, stirring occasionally, 3-4 minutes or until vegetables are crisply tender. Remove vegetables from pan; drain well. Set aside.

2. Pour liquid egg whites into same pan. Cook over medium-low heat, lifting edge of egg whites and pulling them toward center while lifting pan to allow uncooked egg to cover pan. Repeat as needed 1-2 minutes or until egg white mixture is set.

3. Sprinkle with bell pepper mixture and 1/4 cup shredded cheese; fold

omelet in half. Place onto serving plate; sprinkle with additional shredded cheese, if desired.

Balsamic Brussels Sprouts with Almond-Encrusted Seared Tuna
INGREDIENTS
For the Brussels sprouts:
- 1½ pounds Brussels sprouts, trimmed and split
- ¼ cup coconut oil
- 1 tablespoon thick balsamic vinegar
- Sea salt and black pepper to taste

For the tuna:
- 3 tuna steaks
- Crushed almonds
- Sea salt to taste
- Pepper to taste
- 2 tablespoons coconut oil

DIRECTIONS
To prepare Brussels sprouts, add coconut oil to a saucepan and turn heat to medium-high. When the oil melts, add the Brussels sprouts, salt, and pepper, then mix. Cover, reduce heat to low, and let cook for 15 minutes.

Add the balsamic vinegar to the pan and stir. Cover and cook on low for 10 more minutes, until Brussels sprouts are tender.

To make the tuna, crush the almonds using a food processor or rolling pin. Salt and pepper the tuna steaks. Press each tuna steak into the crushed almonds to coat, then flip and repeat on the other side.

In a large frying pan, heat the coconut oil until melted and clear. Place tuna steaks in the pan and sear for 2 minutes. Flip and continue to cook for another 2 minutes. Remove the steaks from the pan and slice into strips. Serve with the Brussels sprouts.

Beef and Broccoli Stir Fry
INGREDIENTS
- 1 tablespoon canola oil
- 2 cups broccoli, blanched
- ½ cup thinly sliced carrot
- ½ cup onion, cut into wedges
- 6 ounces sirloin steak, boneless and cut into strips
- 1½ tablespoons chicken broth
- 1 tablespoon low-sodium soy sauce
- ½ teaspoon guar gum or cornstarch
- ¼ teaspoon Splenda sugar substitute
- 1/8 teaspoon salt (optional)

DIRECTIONS
Heat the oil in a large skillet. Add the broccoli, carrot, and onion and cook, stirring frequently, until the vegetables are tender-crisp. Stir in the beef and cook until it reaches desired doneness.

Stir together the chicken broth, soy sauce, guar gum, Splenda, and salt in a small bowl. Add to the beef and vegetables and cook, stirring constantly until the sauce thickens, about 2 to 3 minutes.

Flank Steak Salad with Chimichurri Dressing
INGREDIENT
- 1 large bunch fresh Italian parsley
- 2 tablespoons fresh oregano leaves
- 3 garlic cloves, peeled
- ½ cup olive oil
- ¼ cup red wine vinegar
- 1 teaspoon chipotle hot pepper sauce
- 1½ pounds flank steak
- 8 ounces mixed baby greens
- 12-ounce container marinated small fresh mozzarella balls, drained

DIRECTION
Prepare barbecue (medium-high heat). Combine parsley (with stems), oregano, and garlic in processor; blend 10 seconds. Add ½ cup oil, vinegar, and hot pepper sauce; blend until almost smooth. Season dressing to taste with salt and pepper.

Brush grill rack with oil. Sprinkle steak on both sides with salt and pepper. Grill steak to desired doneness, about 5 minutes per side for medium-rare. Transfer steak to work surface; let rest 5 minutes.

Meanwhile, toss greens in large bowl with some dressing. Transfer to large platter. Sprinkle mozzarella over.

Thinly slice steak across grain on slight diagonal. Arrange steak atop greens. Drizzle with remaining dressing.

Roasted Asparagus
INGREDIENTS
150 grams of fresh asparagus
½ tbsp olive oil
¼ tbsp balsamic vinegar
¼ clove garlic
sea salt and black pepper to taste
cooking spray

DIRECTION
Preheat oven to 450. Break off the woody stems from asparagus. Rinse well.

Toss spears in oil, vinegar and garlic. Season with salt & pepper. lace in shallow baking dish, sprayed. Bake for 6-10 minutes.

Chicken Zucchini Poppers
INGREDIENTS
1 lb. ground chicken breast

2 Cups grated zucchini (leave peel on)
2-3 green onions, sliced
3-4 TBSP cilantro, minced
1 Clove garlic, minced
1 TSP salt
1/2 TSP pepper

DIRECTIONS
1. Mix ground chicken and remaining ingredients in large mixing bowl.

2. Grab a frying pan or skillet and grease with olive oil. From the bowl spoon out 8-10 nugget sized pieces onto the skillet.

3. Over medium heat cook the chicken poppers for five minutes on each side.

4. You can eat plain or serve with your favorite dip or sauce.

Breakfast "Souffle"
INGREDIENTS
4 egg whites well beaten with salt, pepper, and random seasonings
-sauteed chopped veggies in oil.

DIRECTIONS
Put all of it in a square baking pan - sprayed with non-stick spray - and baked on 400 for about 20 minutes - until the center stops being jiggly.

At the end, top it with 5 oz of shredded cheese and pop back in the oven long enough to let it melt.

Kale and Sweet Potato Sauté
INGREDIENTS
- 2 cups cubed and peeled sweet potatoes, cut into ¼-inch cubes (about 1 large or 2 medium)

- 1 Tbsp. coconut oil
- ½ cup thinly sliced red onion (about ½ small onion)
- 2 cloves garlic, minced
- 4 cups kale, tightly-packed, washed and torn with tough stems removed (about 1 bunch)
- Sea salt and pepper to taste
- Lemon wedges, optional

Creamy Garlic Spaghetti Squash Casserole
INGREDIENTS
- 1 medium spaghetti squash
- 4 cups broccoli florets
- 1 lb sausage (spicy Italian or Chorizo are excellent choices)
- 2 cups mushrooms, diced
- 1/4 cup arrowroot flour
- 2 tbsp minced garlic
- 16 oz coconut milk
- Salt and pepper (about 1 tsp each)

DIRECTIONS
- Preheat oven to 425 degrees fahrenheit.

- Slice the spaghetti squash lengthwise and scoop out the seeds. Place the two halves face-down on a baking sheet and place in the oven to bake for 30 minutes.

- While the squash is cooking, get the sausage going. Heat a large pan over medium heat and add in the sausage. Break it into pieces with a spatula and cook, stirring occasionally, until browned and cooked through, about 8 minutes. Remove from pan and set aside. Reserve at least 1 tbsp of fat in the pan for the sauce you'll make later.

- Remove squash from oven after 30 minutes and set aside to cool. Keep the oven on at 425 degrees.

- While the squash is cooling, prepare the creamy garlic sauce. Heat the same pan you cooked the sausage in over medium heat. Once hot, add mushrooms and cook until they begin to soften, about 2 minutes. Add in the arrowroot flour and minced garlic and stir around to mix well with the mushrooms, about 1-2 minutes.

- Next, add in coconut milk, stirring constantly for 2 minutes. Be sure to mix well to dissolve all of the flour into the milk (you don't want any flour clumps). Use a whisk to mix if needed. The sauce will bubble and thicken, keep stirring to prevent burning. After 2 minutes turn heat down to low and simmer. Stir in salt and pepper.

- Now, put it all together. With a fork, scrape out the spaghetti squash "noodles" into a medium casserole dish. Add the cooked sausage, broccoli, and creamy garlic sauce. Mix everything together well.

- Place back in the oven to bake for 15 more minutes. Remove and serve

Breakfast Sausage
INGREDIENTS
- 2 teaspoons dried sage
- 2 teaspoons salt
- 1 teaspoon ground black pepper
- 1/4 teaspoon dried marjoram
- 1 tablespoon brown sugar
- 1/8 teaspoon crushed red pepper flakes
- 1 pinch ground cloves
- 2 pounds ground pork

DIRECTIONS
1. In a small, bowl, combine the sage, salt, ground black pepper, marjoram, brown sugar, crushed red pepper and cloves. Mix well.

2. Place the pork in a large bowl and add the mixed spices to it. Mix well with your hands and form into patties.

3. Saute the patties in a large skillet over medium high heat for 5 minutes per side, or until internal pork temperature reaches 160 degrees F (73 degrees C).

Turkey burger stuffed with Zuchinni/mushrooms
INGREDIENTS
- 4 ozs of 94% or more lean ground turkey
- 1/2 cup of the following diced veggies:
- Zuchinni & Mushrooms (I used white button)
- 3T shredded carrots
- 1 tablespoon dehydrated onions
- 1 teaspoon onion powder
- .5 teaspoon garlic powder
- .5 teaspoon coarse black pepper
- Salt to taste

DIRECTIONS

Finely dice your veggies and put in a large bowl... add your ground turkey and your seasonings and mix well by hand, all the ingredients and shape into a patty. Some of the veggies will fall out, so press the loose ones on top of the formed patty.

Spray a skillet with canola or safflower oil and heat, using medium/low; the burger will be very large and you don't want to cook it too fast. When heated, add your burger and cook until brown and firm and turn over, and cook until done.

Internal temperature should be 165 degrees.

Serve on a hamburger bun, pita pocket, flavored tortilla, with lettuce, tomatos, etc, or alone with a salad.

Porterhouse Steaks with Compound Butter

INGREDIENTS

For the Compound Butter:
- 1 stick unsalted butter, softened
- 1 clove garlic, peeled
- 3 tablespoons fresh thyme leaves
- Zest of 1 lemon
- 1/2 teaspoon salt
- Dash of cayenne

For the Porterhouse Steaks:
- 4 Porterhouse Steaks, 1 - 1 1/4 inch thick
- Hot Smoked Paprika
- Salt and Pepper

DIRECTIONS

1. Place all the ingredients for the compound butter in a food processor. Puree until smooth and creamy. Scoop the compound butter onto wax paper and roll into a cylinder. Wrap the ends under and refrigerate.

2. For the Porterhouse Steaks: Heat the grill to high heat. Generously sprinkle with salt, pepper, and smoked paprika. Grill for 2-4 minutes per side, to desired interior color. 2 minutes per side for medium-rare.

3. Once off the grill, tent the steaks with foil and allow them to rest 10 minutes before serving. Slice the compound butter and top each warm steak with a slice.

Creamy Salsa Verde Chicken Skillet

INGREDIENTS
- 1 1/2 - 2 pounds boneless skinless chicken breast cutlets (chicken breast cut into thin pieces)

- 1 tablespoon butter
- 2 garlic cloves, minced
- 16 ounce jar tomatilla salsa verde
- 1 cup chicken broth
- 4 ounces low fat cream cheese
- 1/2 cup chopped cilantro
- Salt and pepper

DIRECTIONS
1. Place a large skillet over medium heat. Add the butter and once melted, add the chicken breast cutlets. Salt and pepper liberally. Sear the chicken for 3-4 minutes per side. Then remove the chicken from the skillet and set aside.

2. In the same skillet, sauté the garlic for 1-2 minutes. Pour in the salsa verde, chicken broth, and add the cream cheese. Whisk the mixture until the cream cheese melts, and the sauce comes together smoothly.

3. Once the sauce is smooth and creamy, add the chicken breasts back to the skillet, along with the cilantro. Warm and flip for 3-5 minutes. Serve the chicken covered in the creamy salsa verde pan sauce.

Market Bean Salad
INGREDIENTS
- 1 pound raw or frozen black eyed peas
- 1/2 pound raw or frozen white acre peas (field peas)
- 1/2 pound mixed sprouted peas and lentils
- 1 pint ripe cherry tomatoes
- 1/2 small red onions, chopped
- 2 garlic cloves, minced
- 1/3 cup chopped flat leaf parsley
- 2 tablespoons apple cider vinegar

- 1/4 cup extra virgin olive oil
- Salt and pepper

DIRECTIONS
1. Place a large pot of water over high heat and bring to a boil. Salt the water liberally, then add the black eyed peas. Simmer for 10 minutes, then add the white acre peas and simmer another 20-30 minutes, until both are soft and tender. Drain the peas in a colander and rinse under cold water to bring the temperature down. Shake to remove excess water.

2. Place the cooked peas (beans) in a large mixing bowl. Add the sprouted peas, red onion, garlic, parsley, vinegar and oil. Toss, then salt and pepper to taste and toss again.

3. Cut the large cherry tomatoes in half and leave the small tomatoes whole. When ready to serve, pour the bean salad out on a serving platter the top with the cherry tomatoes.

Jamaican Jerk Chicken Salad
INGREDIENTS
For the Jamaican Jerk Chicken:
- 2 pounds boneless skinless chicken thighs
- 2-4 habanero peppers, seeded
- 2 tablespoons fresh thyme leaves
- 1/2 small red onion
- 1 tablespoon fresh grated ginger
- 4 garlic cloves
- 3 tablespoons soy sauce
- 2 tablespoons lime juice
- 2 tablespoons brown sugar
- 2 teaspoons ground allspice
- 1 teaspoon cinnamon
- 1/2 teaspoon nutmeg

- 1 teaspoon salt
- 1/2 teaspoon black pepper

For the Salad:
- 2 heads of romaine lettuce, chopped
- 2 large red bell peppers, seeded and cut into rings
- 2 ripe avocados, peeled and sliced
- 1 english cucumber, sliced
- 1/2 ripe pineapple, cut into chunks
- 1 bottle Honey Mustard Lite Dressing

DIRECTIONS

1. For the Jamaican Jerk Chicken: Place all the ingredients, except the chicken, in the food processor and puree until smooth. (If you are sensitive to spicy heat, use only 1-2 habanero peppers.) Pour the marinade into a large zip bag and add the chicken. Allow the chicken to marinate for at least one hour, but up to 16 hours.

2. When the chicken is ready to grill, preheat the grill to medium heat. Once hot, remove the chicken from the marinade and place on the grill. Grill for 5 minutes per side. Then allow the chicken to rest 5 minutes before cutting.

3. Meanwhile, grill the red pepper rings for 1-2 minutes per side to soften.

4. Once the chicken has rested, cut into strips. Arrange the romaine lettuce on a large platter, topped with grilled peppers, cucumbers, pineapple and avocado slices. Fan the chicken pieces over the top and drizzle with Newman's Own Honey Mustard Lite Dressing. Serve immediately.

Steak Salad with A1 Vinaigrette
INGREDIENTS
For the Steak Salad:

- 1 large 1 1/2 inch thick ribeye steak (1 1/2 pounds)
- 1 head romaine lettuce
- 3 ripe tomatoes, various colors
- 1 ripe avocado
- 3/4 cup french fried onions (like Frenchs)
- Salt and pepper

For the A1 Vinaigrette:
- 1/4 cup olive oil
- 1/4 cup sour cream
- 1/4 cup A1 Steak Sauce
- 2 tablespoons red wine vinegar
- 2 tablespoons honey

DIRECTIONS

1. Preheat the grill to high heat. Salt and pepper the ribeye steak on both sides. Once the grill is hot, place the steak on it and grill for 3-4 minutes per side.

2. Meanwhile, place all the ingredients for the A1 Vinaigrette in a glass jar. Screw the lid on tight and shake until smooth and thick. Salt and pepper to taste.

3. Roughly chop the romaine lettuce and place on a large platter. Slice the avocado and arrange over the lettuce. Then cut the tomatoes into wedges and arrange over the salad as well.

4. Slice the grilled steak against the grain. Fan the sliced steak over the salad and sprinkle fried onions over the top. Then drizzle the steak salad with A1 Vinaigrette and serve.

Roasted Harvest Vegetables
INGREDIENTS
- 1/2 teaspoon rubbed sage
- 1 teaspoon season salt

- 1/2 teaspoon black pepper
- 3 tablespoons olive oil
- 1/2 teaspoon Ground Nutmeg
- 2 cups cut-up red potatoes, 1-inch chunks
- 1 1/2 cups cut-up carrots, 1-inch chunks
- 1 1/2 cups cut-up red onions, 1-inch chunks
- 1 1/2 cups cut-up butternut squash, 1-inch chunks
- 1 1/2 cups cut-up parsnips, 1-inch chunks

DIRECTIONS
1. Preheat oven to 450°F. Mix seasoned salt, pepper, nutmeg and sage in small bowl. Toss vegetables with oil in large bowl. Sprinkle seasoning mixture over vegetables; toss to coat well.

2. Spread vegetables in single layer on foil-lined 15x10x1-inch baking pan.

3. Bake 30 to 35 minutes or until vegetables are tender and golden brown.

Baked Sweet Potato Chips
INGREDIENTS
- 1 1/2 pounds sweet potatoes
- 1/3 cup olive oil and salt

DIRECTIONS
1. Preheat the oven to 400 degrees F. Line several baking sheets with parchment paper and set aside. Use a slicer to cut the sweet potatoes into paper-thin rounds. (I set mine to the thinnest setting.) You can use a knife to do this, but it takes much longer.

2. Pile all the sweet potato rounds into a large bowl and pour the olive oil over the top. Gently toss to coat every piece with oil. Then lay the sweet potato rounds out on the baking sheets in a single layer.

3. Sprinkle the chips lightly with Diamond Crystal® Kosher Salt. Bake for 20-25 minutes until crisp and golden around the edges. Remove from the oven and cool for 5 minutes on the baking sheets. Then move the chips to a bowl, or plastic bag to store. If you happen to find a few chips with soft centers, pop them back in the oven for about 5 minutes.

Greek Chicken Salad Sandwiches

INGREDIENTS

- 1 cups chopped cooked chicken (use leftover grilled chicken or a rotisserie chicken)
- ½ cups chopped cucumber
- ½ cups halved red grapes
- ½ cup low fat plain greek yogurt
- ½ cup finely chopped scallions
- 1 tablespoons capers, drained
- ½ tablespoon fresh chopped dill
- ½ tablespoon fresh chopped parsley
- 1 teaspoons honey
- 2 garlic cloves, minced
- Zest of one lemon
- Salt and pepper
- 1 Loaf Saaa-Wheat Bread
- 2 ounces alfalfa sprouts

DIRECTIONS

1. Chop all ingredients in preparation. Place the chopped chicken, cucumber, grapes, yogurt, scallions, capers, dill, parsley, honey, garlic, and lemon zest in a large bowl. Mix well.

2. Sprinkle 1 teaspoon salt and 1/2 teaspoon ground pepper over the chicken salad and mix well. Taste, then add more salt and pepper if needed.

3. Scoop the chicken salad onto slices of eureka!® Organic Saaa-Wheat Bread. Top with alfalfa sprouts and another slice of bread.

Brown Sugar Baked Salmon and Vegetables
INGREDIENTS
- 2 pound whole salmon fillet
- 3 medium yellow squash, thinly sliced
- 2 medium zucchini, thinly sliced
- 2 tablespoons olive oil
- 1 teaspoons kosher salt
- 1/2 teaspoon ground black pepper
- 1/4 cup packed dark brown sugar
- 1 1/2 teaspoons stone ground mustard

DIRECTIONS
1. Preheat the oven to 425 degrees F. Line a rimmed baking sheet with parchment paper or foil.

2. Place the salmon, skin side down, on the baking sheet.

3. Arrange the vegetables alongside the salmon around the edges of the baking sheet. Drizzle the vegetables with olive oil. Sprinkle the salmon and vegetables with salt and pepper. Cover the fish and vegetables with another piece of parchment paper or foil. Bake for 10 minutes.

4. Meanwhile in a small bowl, combine the brown sugar and stone ground mustard. Remove the salmon from the oven and remove the top piece of parchment paper. Spread the brown sugar mixture over the top of the salmon. Place the pan back in the oven and bake until the thickest part reaches 135 degrees F, about 15 minutes.

Wild Mushroom and Goat Cheese Frittata
INGREDIENTS

- 8 large eggs
- ½ cup whole milk
- 3 tablespoons vegetable oil
- 4 ounces sliced wild mushrooms, sliced (crimini, oyster, shitake…)
- 1 large shallot, quartered and sliced
- 1 small clove garlic, minced
- 6-8 drops of truffle oil (optional)
- ¾ cup chopped zucchini
- 3 ounces soft goat cheese
- ¼ cup chopped green onions
- Salt and Pepper
- Oil

DIRECTIONS

1. Preheat oven to 350 degrees F. Preheat a skillet to medium-high. Add 1 tablespoon oil to the hot skillet, then add shallot. Sauté for 2 minutes. Then add the garlic and toss.

2. Add the sliced mushrooms. Carefully add the truffle oil, if desired. Sauté the mushrooms for 5-10 minutes, until deep brown, to render out the moisture. Finally, add the zucchini to the skillet and sauté another 2-3 minutes. *Truffle oil is potent; use it sparingly.

3. Transfer the veggies to a plate and wipe the skillet with a paper towel. Put the skillet back over high heat with 2 tablespoons oil. Mix eggs and milk with ½ teaspoon salt and 1/4 teaspoon fresh pepper. Whisk until frothy.

4. Briskly swirl the skillet around as you pour the egg mixture in. This creates a crust on the outer edge. Then add the mushroom and zucchini mixture back to the skillet and crumble the goat cheese over the top.

5. Remove from heat and place in the oven for 15-20 minutes until cooked

through. Slide out of pan onto a cutting board and cut into wedges.

Slow Cooker Black Bean Soup Recipe
INGREDIENTS
For the Black Bean Soup Recipe:
- 1 pound dried black beans, rinsed
- 1 large onion, peeled and diced
- 2 medium red bell peppers, seeded and diced
- 2 quarts vegetable broth
- 1/3 cup Franks Cayenne Hot Sauce
- 6 garlic cloves, minced
- 2 bay leaves
- 1 tablespoon ground cumin
- Salt and Pepper

Possible Toppings:
- Chopped scallions
- Cilantro
- Jalapeno slices
- Shredded cheese
- Lime wedges
- Sour cream (or plain yogurt)

DIRECTIONS
1. Place all the ingredients in a slow cooker and season with 1 teaspoon of salt and 1/2 teaspoon ground pepper. Turn the slow cooker on medium, cover, and cook for 10-12 hours. (You could soak the beans in water overnight to reduce the cooking time by half, but it's not necessary.)

2. Once the beans are tender, remove the bay leaves. Use an immersion blender to blend the soup until two-thirds of the beans are pureed and the soup is thick. Salt and pepper to taste, then serve warm with fresh toppings.

Mesir Wat Red Lentil Stew with Ayib

INGREDIENTS

For the Red Lentil Stew:

- ½ cups red lentils
- ½ large onion, chopped
- 1 tablespoons butter
- ½ tablespoons fresh grated ginger
- ½ cloves, garlic, minced
- ½ tablespoon smoked paprika
- ½ teaspoon tumeric
- ½ teaspoon garam masala
- 1 tablespoons tomato paste
- Salt and pepper

For the Ayib (Iab):

- 1 cups (12 ounces) small curb cottage cheese
- Zest of 1 lemon
- 1 tablespoons plain greek yogurt
- 1/4 teaspoon salt

DIRECTIONS

1. Place a large sauce pot over medium heat. Add the butter and chopped onions and saute for 3-5 minutes, until soft. Add the ginger and garlic and saute another 2 minutes.

2. Next add the spices and tomato paste along with 2 teapoons of salt. Mix well, then add the lentils and 6 cups of water.

3. Cover the pot and bring to a boil. Once boiling, lower the heat and simmer for 20 minutes.

4. Uncover and stir the lentils, then continue to cook uncovered for another 10-15 minutes until a thick porridge-like consistency is reached. Remove from heat and cover until ready to serve.

5. For the Ayib: Rinse and drain the cottage cheese in cold water until only clean curds are left. Place the curds in a bowl and press them dry with paper towels until most of the moisture in removed and the curds have broken up.

6. Mix in the yogurt, lemon zest and salt. Refrigerated until ready to serve. To serve: Scoop the Mesir Wat into bowl and place a generous dollop of Ayib on top.

Zucchini and Green Chutney Salad
INGREDIENTS
For the Green Chutney:
• ¼ cup chana dal (similar to yellow lentils)
• 1 cup water, divided
• 1-2 serrano peppers, seeded
• 1 ½ tablespoons lime juice
• 3 cloves garlic, roughly chopped
• 1 bunch cilantro, stems and all
• 1 tablespoon sugar
• 1 teaspoon salt

For the Zucchini Salad:
• 4 zucchinis
• 1 large mango
• ½ red onion

DIRECTIONS
1. Preheat the oven to 450 degrees F. Place the Chana Dal on a baking sheet and roast for 5-10 minutes, until golden brown.

2. Then move the Chana Dal to the food processor with a ¼ cup of water and puree until smooth. Add a little extra water if needed.

3. Add the serrano pepper, lime juice, garlic, cilantro sugar and salt. Pulse to break down. Then add the remaining water and puree until

smooth. Blend in the sugar and salt and pulse to mix. (Makes about 2 cups.)

4. Using a veggie peeler, slice the zucchinis into long ribbons and place them in a serving bowl. Peel and slice the mango into thin strips. Slice the onion into thin slivers. Top the zucchini with mango and red onion and drizzle with green chutney.

Easy Breakfast Omelet

This is a great and healthy way to start your day. Eggs are among the richest sources of protein and these are inexpensive, too. Make a high-carb breakfast by mixing in fruits, whole grain toast, or oatmeal. You can prepare this for lunch or dinner and change the ratios depending on whether you are on a high-carb or low-carb day.

Ingredients:
4 egg whites
1 medium onion, chopped
1 medium bell pepper, chopped
Mushrooms, chopped
1 medium tomato, chopped
Spinach
Olive oil in spray bottle
A dash of salt and pepper or low –sodium seasoning blend

Note: You can make use of any other filling that you like. This makes 1 serving, if you want more, double the portions accordingly.
Procedure:
1. In a small bowl, whisk the egg whites for at least 45 seconds.
2. Add the vegetables and mix.
3. Spray olive oil on a non-stick pan and set to medium to high heat.
4. Add the egg whites and the veggie mixture into the pan. Season.
5. Let the omelet to finish cooking on one side and flip over to the other side with a spatula, to let it cook.

Healthy and Delicious Burrito

Ingredients:
- 6 egg whites
- 4 tbsp ground turkey
- 2 handfuls spinach
- 2-4 leaves romaine lettuce
- 2 tbsp salsa
- Vegetable oil in spray bottle
- A dash of salt and pepper

Note: This makes 2 servings, double the recipe if you want more.
Procedure:
1. Spray oil in a non-stick pan and set to medium heat.
2. Cook turkey in oil. Set aside.
3. In a large mixing bowl, beat egg whites.
4. Using another non-stick pan, spray vegetable oil and set to medium to high heat. Cook the egg in the pan. As the egg begins to set, add in the turkey and spinach. Season. Let it cook further.
5. When cooked, wrap the turkey, egg and spinach combo in two or four leaves of romaine lettuce.
6. Garnish with the salsa and roll it up.

Low-Carb Breakfast Tacos

Ingredients:
- 4 egg whites
- Corn tortillas
- 3 tomatoes, sliced
- 3 tbsp salsa
- A dash of low-sodium spice blend
- Oil in spray bottle

Note: This recipe makes 1 serving, double if you want to or adjust ingredients according to what you need.

Procedure:
1. Spray oil onto a non-stick pan. Set to medium heat.
2. Whisk the egg whites.
3. Season with the spice blend.
4. Cook until you get your preferred "scrambled" consistency.
5. Serve with corn tortillas.
6. Add in salsa and tomato slices.

Delicious Breakfast Burrito
Ingredients:
- 1 tsp canola oil
- ¼ cup onions, chopped
- 2 egg whites, whisked
- 1 low-carb high fiber tortilla
- A pinch of salt
- A pinch of pepper
- Salsa

Note: This makes 1 serving of breakfast burrito. Adjust portions accordingly.
Procedure:
- Set a non-stick pan to medium heat and cook the onions until soft.
- Season with salt and pepper.
- Add in beaten egg whites. Cook until almost set. Set aside.
- Warm tortilla in a dry pan. Pour in cooked eggs on top of the tortilla.
- Add salsa.
- Roll up and eat.

High-Carb Egg Muffin Special
Ingredients:
- 8 egg whites
- 4 slices of tomatoes
- 2 toasted English muffins
- A dash of low-sodium spice blend

Note: This recipe is good for a double-serving, add portions accordingly if you want to make more.

Procedure:

1. Whisk egg whites in a mixing bowl.
2. Spray oil in a non-stick pan. Set over medium to high heat.
3. Add the beaten eggs to the pan. Cook.
4. Add the sliced tomatoes and cooked eggs on the toasted muffin.
5. Season.

Your Favourite Breakfast Ham Omelet

Ingredients:

- 3 egg whites, whisked
- 2 tbsp low-sodium ham, chopped
- 1 tbsp onions, chopped
- 1 tbsp green bell pepper, chopped
- 1 tbsp tomato, sliced
- Fresh salsa
- A portion of cheddar cheese
- A dash of salt and pepper or low-sodium spice blend

Note: This makes 1 serving, you can double the portions if you want to make it for two persons.

Procedure:

1. Heat a non-stick pan to medium-high.
2. Add the beaten egg whites. Season.
3. Let the egg whites set on one side.
4. Place the ham, onions, bell peppers and tomatoes in the middle and continue cooking. Fold in half to enclose filling.
5. Add salsa and cheese before serving.

A Healthy BLT Sandwich

This is perfect for an anytime of the day meal as it is easy to prepare. It's ready in minutes so if you are late for work or an appointment, this will be great to perk up your day.

Ingredients:
- 2 wheat bread slices, toasted
- 2 medium tomatoes, sliced
- 2oz lean turkey breast
- 2 turkey bacon, cooked
- 2 green lettuce leaves

Note: This recipe is good for one, adjust accordingly.

Procedure:
1. Simply layer the meats, tomato slices, and lettuce between the toast and you're good to go.

Healthy Mini Egg Omelet

Ingredients:
- 4 cups broccoli
- 4 whole eggs
- 1 cup egg whites
- ¼ cup low-fat cheddar cheese, shredded
- ¼ cup pecorino Romano cheese, shredded
- Salt and pepper to taste
- Cooking spray

Note: This recipe makes 4 mini omelets. Double the portions if you need more.

Procedure:
1. Preheat oven to 350°.
2. Steam the broccoli in water for 6 to 7 minutes. When cooked, crush into smaller pieces.
3. Add olive oil and season with salt and pepper.
4. Spray a standard non-stick cupcake molder with cooking spray and put broccoli mixture evenly into 9 molds.
5. In a mixing bowl, beat whole eggs, egg whites and grated pecorino Romano cheese. Add salt and pepper to taste. Pour over the broccoli mixture until mold is ¾ full.

6. Top each with grated cheddar cheese.
7. Bake for at least 20 minutes.
8. Serve immediately. If you have leftovers, wrap them in plastic wrap or put in a zip-lock plastic bag and refrigerate. It is good for one week.

Special Breakfast Enchilada
Ingredients:
- 3 cups egg whites (from about 18 large eggs)
- 2 tbsp water
- Salt and pepper to taste
- Cooking spray
- 1 tsp olive oil
- ½ cup chopped scallions
- 1 medium diced tomatoes
- 2 tbsp chopped cilantro
- 10 oz pack frozen spinach
- 4.5 oz can chopped green chilis
- Salt and pepper to taste
- ½ cup grated cheese
- 1 cup green enchilada sauce
- 1 medium avocado, diced

Note: This recipe yields 6 servings.
Procedure:
1. Preheat oven to350°F.
2. Pour in 1/ cup enchilada sauce on the bottom of a baking dish (9x12 inches).
3. In a mixing bowl, beat egg whites, add water, and a pinch of salt and pepper.
4. Coat a non-stick pan with cooking spray and set stove to medium heat.
5. Add ½ cup of the egg whites, swirl evenly to cover the entire pan. Cook for about 2 minutes and then flip to cook the other side. Set

aside and repeat with the remaining egg whites. You should be able to make 6 "egg tortillas".

6. Heat oil in another non-stick pan and set to medium heat. Cook the scallions for about 2 to 3 minutes. Add tomato and cilantro. Add salt and pepper to taste and cook for another 1 minute. Add in spinach and green chili and let it cook for another 5 minutes. Adjust seasoning according to your preference.

7. Remove from heat and add ½ cup of cheese and mix well.

8. Divide spinach among the "egg tortillas". Roll up and place each side down in the baking dish. Top the "tortillas" with your remaining enchilada sauce and cheese. Cover the baking dish with foil and bake until cheese is melted, which will take about 20 to 25 minutes.

9. You can serve topped with diced scallions and avocados.

Bacon-Wrapped Mini Meatloaf

Ingredients:
- 1 lb lean ground beef
- ½ lb bacon, cut in chunks
- 8 strips of bacon (do not cut)
- ¼ cup coconut milk
- 2 cloves minced garlic
- ½ cup minced fresh chives
- Chopped, fresh parsley
- Ground black pepper

Note: This recipe serves 4 people.

Procedure:
1. Preheat oven to 400°F.
2. In a mixing bowl, mix ground beef, bacon chunks, garlic, chives, and coconut milk. Season with ground black pepper. Bacon replaces salt.
3. Put one bacon slice each on a medium-sized muffin molder, creating rings.

4. Fill the rings with the mixed beef.
5. Cook in the oven for about 30 minutes.
6. Remove the mini meatloaf and top with parsley.
7. This is a good low-carb day breakfast.

Low-Carb Egg Benedict Breakfast
Ingredients:
- 2 tbsp butter
- 1 beaten egg
- 1 slice ham
- Lazy hollandaise sauce

For Hollandaise Sauce
- ¼ cup mayonnaise
- 1 tsp lemon or lime juice
- ¼ tsp pepper

Note: This recipe is good for one; adjust if serving 2 or more.
Procedure:
1. In a small non-stick skillet, heat butter and add egg. Allow the egg to form into a solid mass; if you have an "egg ring", it is perfect for this. Flip to cook the other side.
2. Let the egg cool for about 2 to 3 minutes.
3. With the use of a regular drinking glass or a circle cookie cutter, cut the ham to fit the scrambled eggs' diameter. You might need to fold the cooked egg several times to create a layer.
4. Cut the cooked egg to look like a muffin and place on top of the ham.
5. Top with hollandaise sauce.

How to Make Hollandaise Sauce
1. Blend all the ingredients for the sauce. Heat before topping onto your egg Benedict.

Avocado Grilled Chicken with Mango Salad

Ingredients:
- 1 lb chicken breast
- 1 cup avocado, diced
- 1 cup mango, diced (1 ½ mangoes)
- 2 tbsp red onion, diced
- 6 cups baby red lettuce

For the Vinaigrette
- 2 tbsp olive oil
- 2 tbsp balsamic vinegar
- Salt and pepper

Procedure:
1. Grill chicken breasts and slice lengthwise. Put in a salad bowl.
2. Whisk together the ingredients for the vinaigrette and set aside.
3. Toss avocado, mango, red onion and sliced chicken breasts.
4. Line a salad platter with the baby lettuce and place the avocado and chicken mixture.
5. Drizzle with the vinaigrette just before serving.
6. This low-carb chicken salad is not just perfect for breakfast but also for lunch and dinner.

Chapter 8: Lunch + Dinner Recipes

3-Flavor Chicken

Ingedients:

- 2 chicken breasts
- Olive oil in a spray bottle
- Baby spinach leaves, blanched
- 1 medium tomato, sliced
- 2 tsp each of tomato, basil, and garlic seasoning

Note: This recipe makes 2 portions; you can double the ingredients to make 4, and so on.

Procedure:

1. Season chicken breasts on both sides.
2. Set a non-stick pan to medium heat and spray olive oil.
3. Add the seasoned chicken breasts and cook on each side.
4. Serve with tomatoes and spinach. You may also sprinkle some oil or seasoning on the veggies.
5. Another option is to season with balsamic vinegar.

Chicken Caribbean

Ingredients:

- 2 chicken breasts (skinless)
- Olive oil in a spray bottle
- 1 tsp low sodium soy sauce
- 1 tsp cider vinegar
- 1 tbsp Caribbean jerk seasoning
- 1 tsp water

Note: This makes 2 servings, adjust accordingly if you want to make more.

Procedure:

- In a zip-lock bag or a container with cover, place all the ingredients. Massage the chicken gently until it is fully coated with marinade.
- Let the marinated chicken sit for at least 30 to 45 minutes.
- Grill the chicken over medium oil. You can also broil if you want to.
- Serve hot with your veggie salad for low-carb days or brown rice for high-carb days.

For more flavorful chicken, you can marinate overnight. You may also keep it in the refrigerator (if you are making a batch) and cook when needed.

Italian Chicken with Herbs

Ingredients:

- 2 chicken breasts, boneless and skinless
- Olive in spray bottle
- A dash of dried red pepper, ground
- 1/3 tsp salt
- ½ tsp Italian seasoning
- 4 tsp red wine vinegar
- 1 tsp water

Note: This recipe makes 2 portions, double the measurements if you are preparing more.

Procedure:

1. In a zip-lock bag (you can also use a container with cover), place all the ingredients. Make sure the chicken is coated with the marinade. Leave for at least 30 minutes. To make it more flavorful, prepare the day before you intend to cook it and just keep in the refrigerator.
2. Grill chicken over medium to high heat, cooking on each side.
3. For a low-carb day, add in your favorite vegetable salad. You can

also drizzle the chicken with a few drops of salad dressing.

4. For high-carb days, serve with brown rice and a side dish of steamed veggies.

Lime Chicken with Spices

Ingredients:
- 2 chicken breast halves, boneless and skinless
- 2 tsp butter
- 2 tsp olive oil
- 2 tbsp low sodium chicken broth
- 1 ½ tbsp lime juice
- ¼ tsp salt
- ¼ tsp pepper
- ½ tsp garlic powder
- ¼ tsp onion powder
- A pinch of cayenne pepper
- A pinch of paprika
- ¼ tsp thyme

Note: This is good for 2; adjust portioning when you intend to serve more.

Procedure:

1. Mix together the seasonings and the chicken breast in a large zip-lock bag. Make sure that the chicken is well-coated. Let it stand for at least 1 hour to let the flavor set in. If you want to make it more flavorful, marinate the chicken overnight.
2. Set a non-stick skillet to medium heat and put the butter and olive oil.
3. When butter is melted, add in the chicken breasts and cook on each side.
4. Remove from pan and set aside.
5. To the same skillet, add the lime juice and the chicken broth. With the use of a whisk, mix the liquids and continue boiling until sauce is slight reduced.

6. Add the cooked chicken into the skillet and coat with the sauce.
7. Serve with blanched asparagus or broccoli on low-carb days. On the other hand, serve with sweet potatoes on your high-carb days.
8. You may add grated cheese on reward days.

Baked Potatoes and Chicken

This is a complete meal that the whole family will love, whether or not they are also on a diet.

Ingredients:

- 2 chicken breasts, skinless, diced
- 1 lb red potatoes
- Oil in spray bottle
- A bunch of asparagus, trimmed and cut into 1-inch pieces (you can also use red and green bell pepper or any other vegetable you like)
- 1/3 fresh basil, chopped
- 4 gloves of garlic, thinly sliced
- 1 ½ tbsp olive oil
- 1 tsp fresh rosemary, chopped
- A pinch of ground pepper to taste
- ½ cup chicken broth (optional)

Note: This is good for one person only but if you have to prepare for more people, you can adjust measurement accordingly.

Procedure:

1. Preheat oven to 400°.
2. Spray your baking dish with oil and place the chicken breasts, potatoes, tomatoes, vegetables, basil, garlic, olive oil and chicken broth. Sprinkle fresh rosemary and ground pepper.
3. Bake for about 45 minutes, checking and turning occasionally to make sure both sides are cooked.
4. Serve.

High-Carb Chicken and Turkey Medley

Ingredients:

- 2 chicken breasts, boneless and skinless
- 2 slices Turkey bacon slices, diced
- Olive oil in spray bottle
- 1 ½ tsp butter
- ¼ cup apple, diced
- 2 ½ tbsp apple cider
- 1 cup brown rice
- 2 ½ tbsp low-sodium chicken broth
- 1 tsp thyme, dried
- salt and pepper

Note: This recipe serves only 1 person, adjust measurements if preparing for more than 1.

Procedure:

1. Spray oil on a non-stick pan and set to medium heat.
2. Put the chicken breasts to the pan and season with salt and pepper. Cook both sides.
3. Remove cooked chicken from pan and set aside.
4. In the same pan, cook the turkey bacon for about 5 minutes or until it turns brown.
5. Add apple and thyme. Add another pinch of salt and pepper.
6. When the apples turn to brown, bring in the apple cider and chicken broth.
7. Increase to high heat.
8. Let the sauce cook until it thickens, don't forget to stir continuously.
9. Add in butter and let it melt.
10. Next, put back in the pan and coat with the sauce. Simmer for about 2 to 3 minutes.
11. You can serve with brown rice.
12. If you making several batches, you can store in the freezer and simply reheat when needed.

Pork Roast

Ingredients:
- 1 lb pork tenderloin
- 5 gloves of garlic, minced
- 1 tsp dried parsley flakes
- ½ tsp dried thyme leaves
- 1 tsp pepper
- 1 tbsp lemon juice (you can also use lime juice, depending on what's available)
- 1 tsp olive oil

Note: This recipe can serve at least 4 people.

Procedure:
1. Preheat oven at 450°F.
2. Line a roasting pan with foil and spray with oil.
3. In a mixing bowl, combine garlic, parsley, thyme and pepper.
4. In a small cup, put the lemon juice.
5. Brush pork with lemon juice and then rub with the garlic and spice mixture over the top and both its sides. Place in the roasting pan with the garlic and spice marinade side up.
6. Bake for about 35 minutes or until pork is evenly cooked.
7. Let the pork stand for 5 to 10 minutes before cutting and serving.
8. Serve with your favorite vegetable salad.

Healthy Baked Meatballs

Ingredients:
- 16oz ground Turkey meat (93% lean)
- 2 egg whites
- 1/2 cup oatmeal
- ¼ cup nonfat milk
- ½ cup parsley
- 1 tbsp onions, dehydrated flakes
- ½ tsp oregano, ground
- ½ tsp garlic powder

Note: This recipe serves 4 with about 8 meatballs each.

Procedure:

1. Preheat oven at 400°F.
2. Spray a baking dish with oil.
3. In a mixing bowl, combine egg whites, oats and milk. Add in parsley, oregano, onions, garlic power and mix well. Add in ground turkey and mix well.
4. Make about 32 uniform meatballs (about 1 scoop).
5. Line in the baking dish, with a good distance from one another.
6. Bake in the oven for about 7 to 10 minutes or until the inside is cooked.
7. Serve with brown rice for high-carb days or vegetable salad on low-carb days.

Healthy BBQ

Ingredients:

- 1 ¼ lbs boneless pork tenderloin, lean
- Sea salt
- Ground black pepper
- Garlic powder
- ¼ cup and 2 tbsp barbecue sauce (separate)
- Olive oil spray

Note: This BBQ recipe yields 4 servings.

Procedure:

1. Slice pork tenderloin in half, crosswise, and then slice each half lengthwise into quarters, yielding 8 strips. Season slices with sea salt, ground pepper and garlic powder. Place pork in a zip-lock plastic bag. Spoon ¼ cup of BBQ sauce and mix with the pork. Refrigerate overnight.
2. Pre-heat broiler. Line a baking sheet with aluminum foil and lightly spray with oil.
3. Place strips on the baking sheet in a single layer.
4. Broil for 2 to 3 minutes. Flip on the other side and continue to broil

for 2 to 3 minutes more.

5. Serve with the sauce dripping. Serve with brown rice for high-carb days and vegetable salad with light dressing on low-carb days.

Delicious Turkey Burger

Ingredients:

- 8 oz raw ground turkey
- Olive oil in a spray bottle
- 1 tsp minced garlic
- ¼ tsp cayenne pepper
- ½ tsp hot sauce (optional)

Note: This recipe serves two persons; you can adjust measurements as needed.

Procedure:

1. In a mixing bowl, combine the ground turkey with cayenne pepper and garlic. Add in the hot sauce if you want. Make sure the turkey and the seasonings are mixed thoroughly. Form into patties.
2. Spray oil in a non-stick pan and set to medium heat. Cook turkey patties on each side.
3. Serve immediately with carrot and celery sticks for low-carb days and boiled red potatoes on high-carb days.

Healthy Steak Tenderloin

Ingredients:

- 6 oz sirloin steak, lean and boneless
- Olive oil in spray bottle
- ¾ steak seasoning
- 1 tsp parsley flakes
- 1 tsp rosemary flakes

Note: This recipe makes 2 servings, you may add portions if you need more.

Procedures:

1. Spray olive oil on each steak.
2. Sprinkle the steaks with seasoning, parsley and rosemary.
3. Grill steak over high heat. You can also cook in a broiler.
4. Serve hot with your favorite greens with light salad dressing on low-carb days. For high-carb days, you can add baked sweet potato or brown rice; and you can still have the veggies as side dish.

Roasted Beef with Stir-Fry Veggies

Ingredients:
- 6 oz lean sirloin steak, boneless
- Olive oil in spray bottle
- 2 tsp low-sodium soy sauce
- ½ tsp cornstarch
- 1/8 ground ginger
- 1 tsp roasted garlic and bell pepper seasoning
- 1/3 cup assorted veggies (you can use snow peas, broccoli, and bell pepper strips)
- 1/3 cup water

Note: This recipe yields 2 portions, double the measurements if you need to make 4.

Procedure:
1. Cut the sirloin steak into 1/4 –inch strips.
2. In a mixing bowl, put the soy sauce, ginger, roasted garlic and bell pepper seasoning, cornstarch and water. Mix thoroughly and set aside.
3. Heat oil on medium to high setting in a non-stick pan. Add beef slices in small batches and cook each for about 5 minutes.
4. Spray more oil if needed.
5. When all the meat slices are done, cook the veggies in the same pan.
6. Serve with almonds or sliced avocado on your low-carb days or with brown rice on high-carb days.

Low-Carb Blue Cheese Steak

Ingredients:

- 6 oz cube steak
- 1/3 cup blue cheese crumbles
- Olive oil in spray bottle
- Red onion, chopped
- ½ tbsp Salt and pepper

Note: This recipe serves 2, double or triple the portions if you need more.

Procedure:

1. Preheat broiler.
2. Heat a non-stick pan over medium heat and spray oil. Add the seasoned meat and cook on each side.
3. Line the broiler pan with foil and place the steak. Top meat with blue cheese and onion.
4. Broil until cheese melts.
5. Serve with steamed greens.
6. If you are making more portions and you want to freeze until you need them, after pan searing the meat, store in a zip-lock plastic and put in the freezer. In a separate zip-lock bag, put onion and blue cheese and freeze as well. You can broil anytime meat is thawed or you can cook it in a microwave oven; just make sure to top the meat with blue cheese and onion.

Sirloin Steak with Veggies

Ingredients:

- 6 oz lean sirloin steak, boneless
- Olive oil in spray bottle
- 1 cup green beans
- 1 medium tomato, chopped
- ¾ tsp garlic, minced
- Salt and pepper to taste

Note: This recipe can serve 1 to 2 persons, if you need to make more portions, adjust the measurements accordingly.

Procedure:

1. In a non-stick pan spray some oil and set stove to high heat. Add meat and cook on each side. Remove from pan and set aside.
2. Adjust heat to medium and in the same pan, add green beans and sauté for 3 minutes and then add garlic and cook for another one minute. Season with salt and pepper.
3. Add diced tomatoes and cook for a minute.
4. Cover pan and let the tomatoes become saucy, about 3 to 4 minutes.
5. Serve the meat with the vegetables on the side.
6. For low-carb days, add sliced avocado; and for high-carb days, serve with baked potato/ sweet potato or brown rice.

Sweet Pork Tenderloin

Ingredients:
- 6 oz lean pork tenderloin
- 1 tbsp honey
- ½ tbsp vinegar
- ¼ tsp vanilla
- 1/8 tsp paprika
- A dash of ground mustard
- Salt and pepper to taste

Note: This makes 2 servings, adjust accordingly if you need more.

Procedure:

1. Combine honey and other flavorings in a zip-lock bag and mix well.
2. Add the pork tenderloin in the zip-lock bag and coat with the honey glaze all over.
3. Heat a non-stick pan over meat settings and cook pork tenderloin on each side.
4. Serve hot with a portion of pecans and vegetable salad on a low-carb day. On the other hand, you can serve it with baked sweet potato or brown rice and side salad for a high-carb day.

Special Tenderloin with Herbs and Spices
Ingredients:
- 6 oz pork tenderloin, lean
- Olive oil in spray bottle
- ½ tsp paprika
- ¼ tsp dried thyme
- ¼ tsp salt
- 1/8 tsp black pepper

Note: The recipe is good for 2 persons so you can adjust measurements when needed.
Procedure:
1. In a mixing bowl, mix all the flavorings and spices. When thoroughly mixed, sprinkle over the pork tenderloins.
2. Spray oil on a non-stick pan and set to medium heat. Add the pork and cook on each side.
3. Serve with your choice of greens for a low-carb day or sweet potato for a high-carb day.

Herbed Roast Pork with Garlic
Ingredients:
- 6 oz lean pork tenderloins
- Olive oil in spray bottle
- 2 tsp roasted garlic and herb seasoning

Note: This is good for 1 to 2 persons so if you need to feed more, adjust measurements.
Procedure:
1. Season pork with the roasted garlic and herb.
2. Spray oil on a non-stick pan and set to medium heat. Cook the pork tenderloin on each side.
3. This is perfect for a low-carb day when you serve with side salad with olive oil and balsamic dressing. If on a high-carb day, you can

serve with steamed asparagus and brown rice.

Grilled Chicken Wings

Ingredients:
- 4 pieces chicken wings
- Chicken spice mix seasoning
- Broccoli, asparagus, lettuce (or your choice of greens)
- Salsa

Note: This is good for 1 to 2 persons.

Procedure:
1. Preheat oven to 350°F.
2. Generously coat chicken wings with seasoning, making sure they are completely coated.
   Insert chicken wings in the oven and cook until they are golden brown and crunchy.
3. Toss your choice of vegetables and top with salsa.
4. This is good for a low-carb day.

Low-Carb Meatballs Barbecue

Ingredients:
- 1 lb ground pork, lean
- 1 tsp granulated sugar substitute
- 1 tsp paprika
- ½ tsp salt
- ¼ tsp black pepper
- ¼ tsp cayenne pepper
- ½ tsp ground cumin
- ¼ tsp celery salt
- 1 medium-sized egg
- ¼ cup almond flour
- 1 tbsp water

For the BBQ Sauce
- ¼ cup yellow mustard
- 2 tsp hot sauce
- 1 tbsp dried onion flakes
- 3 tbsp granulated sugar substitute
- 2 tbsp apple cider vinegar
- 2 tbsp ketchup
- Salt and pepper to taste

Note: This recipe makes 16 meatballs, 4 meatballs per serving.
Procedure:
1. First, mix all the barbecue sauce ingredients in a saucepan, stir until fully mixed and smooth. Over low heat, simmer sauce for about 8 minutes. Set aside.
2. In a mixing bowl, combine all the ingredients for the meatballs and mix. Form into medium-sized balls, this will give you 16 pieces.
3. In a non-stick skillet, fry meatballs over medium heat. Cooking time is 3 to 4 minutes on each side.
4. Toss the cooked meatballs into the barbecue sauce. Once meatballs are fully coated, spread them on a baking dish lined with parchment paper. Broil for about 2 to 3 minutes.
5. Serve with coleslaw or your favorite greens.

Low-Carb Roasted Turkey
Ingredients:
- 1 whole turkey
- 1 tbsp vegetable oil
- 1 tsp Italian seasoning
- Salt and pepper

Note: This yields at least 18 servings.
Procedure:
1. Preheat your outdoor grill to get medium to high heat.
2. Prepare the turkey. After washing it clean, pat to dry. Turn the

wings back so the neck skin is held in place. Turn the legs to a tucked position.

3. Brush turkey skin with oil. Season both inside and out with the Italian seasoning, salt and pepper.
4. Position the turkey, with the breast side up, on the metal grate inside a large roasting pan. Place the pan on the prepared grill.
5. Cooking time is 2 to 3 hours.
6. Remove from the grill and let it stand for about 15 minutes before carving the turkey.
7. Serve with your favorite greens.

Delicious Salmon Fillet with Herbs and Spices
Ingredients:
- 4 pieces salmon fillet, no bones and skin
- ½ cup melted unsalted butter
- 2 tbsp ground paprika
- 1 tbsp ground cayenne pepper
- 1 tbsp onion powder
- 2 tsp salt
- ½ tsp ground white pepper
- ½ tsp ground black pepper
- ¼ tsp dried thyme
- ¼ tsp dried basil
- ¼ tsp dried oregano

Note: This recipe yields 4 servings.
Procedure:
1. In a mixing bowl, mix the spices: paprika, cayenne pepper, salt, onion powder, white and black pepper, basil, thyme and oregano.
2. Brush each salmon fillet with ¼ of the butter and evenly sprinkle with the mixed spices.
3. Drizzle on each side with half of the remaining butter.
4. Heat a large skillet to high and cook salmon, with the butter side down, until crust is blackened; this will take about 2 to 5 minutes.

5. Turn the fillet and drizzle with the last remaining butter.
6. Continue cooking until crust is blackened. It is ready when fish is flaked when you poke with a fork.

Spicy Pork Tenderloin
Ingredients:
- 6 oz pork tenderloin
- 1 tsp butter
- Olive oil in spray bottle
- ½ tsp paprika
- ¼ dried oregano
- ½ tsp garlic powder
- ½ tsp ground cumin
- ¾ tsp salt
- 1/8 tsp fennel seeds
- A dash of ground cayenne pepper
- ¼ cup chicken broth

Note: This recipe makes 2 servings.
Procedure:
1. In a small mixing bowl, combine all the herbs and spices.
2. Brush half of the spice on one side of the tenderloin.
3. Set non-stick pan to medium heat and add the pork, with the spiced side down. While pork is cooking in that position, sprinkle the rest of the spices on top.
4. Cook on each side until browned.
5. Remove from pan and keep the pork warm.
6. On the same pan, add butter and whisk all the browned bits and spices left in the pan. Turn the heat to medium-high and add the chicken broth. Continue whisking until sauce is reduced by half.
7. Place the pork on a serving plate and drizzle the sauce on top.
8. Serve with your potato salad or baked potato for a high-carb day or your favorite greens for a low-carb day.

Easy Garlic and Herb Shrimp Salad

Ingredients:
- 25 pieces large shrimps, peeled and deveined
- Olive oil in a spray bottle
- 2 tsp roasted garlic and herb seasoning
- Raw baby spinach

Note: This makes 2 servings.

Procedure:
1. Thoroughly season shrimp with roasted garlic and herb mix.
2. Spray oil on a non-stick pan and set to medium heat.
3. Cook shrimp.
4. Serve immediately over a bed of baby spinach. You can toss spinach with balsamic vinegar and olive oil before adding the shrimp.

Perfect Salmon Fillet

Ingredients:
- 8 oz salmon fillet
- ½ tbsp butter
- 1 tbsp Cajun seasoning
- 1 tsp minced garlic
- 2 tbsp balsamic vinegar
- 2 lemon wedges

Note: Makes 2 servings. Add portions to make more.

Procedure:
1. Heat a non-stick pan set at medium heat. Melt butter and add salmon. Cook on each side but you have to be careful because salmon cooks rather quickly. If salmon is overcooked, it becomes dry.
2. Remove fish from pan and keep warm.
3. On the same pan, add in the rest of the butter, then add garlic and Cajun seasoning.
4. Cook for about 2 minutes before adding the balsamic vinegar.

Simmer for another 2 minutes, with continuous stirring.

5. Put back the salmon to the pan and finish the cooking process.
6. Place the fillet on a serving plate and garnish with lemon wedges.
7. Serve with steamed asparagus or baby spinach if you are on a low-carb day. When you are on a high-carb day, add brown rice.

Paleo Friendly Meaty Veggie Roll-ups

Yields: 12 roll-ups | Serving Size: 4-6 roll ups |Calories: 71 | Total Fat: 2.0 g | Saturated Fat: 0.6 g | Trans Fat: 0 g | Cholesterol: 29 mg | Sodium: 27 mg | Carbohydrates: 1.2 g | Dietary Fiber: 0 g | Sugars: 0.8 g | Protein: 11.3g | SmartPoints: 1

INGREDIENTS

12 thick slices unprocessed deli meat, we recommend Boar's Head Brand
1 cup sliced vegetables
12 chives, optional

DIRECTIONS

Place desired amount of vegetables on a piece of deli meat. Roll tightly, and if desired, use a chive to tie. Pack in a zip-top plastic bag or airtight container.

Favorite Flavor Combinations:

Roast beef with red bell pepper strips, carrot sticks, and cucumber slices with mustard for dipping.

Chicken with apple slices, red cabbage, and pickle strips with Dijon mustard for dipping.

Turkey with crumbled bacon and sliced avocado with salsa for dipping.

Slow Cooke Lower Carb Cabbage Roll Stew (Be sure to save enough for tomorrow's lunch!)

Yields: 6 Servings | Serving Size: 1 1/3 Cup | Calories: 242 | Fat: 13 g | Carbohydrates: 14 g | Fiber: 3 g | Sugars: 6 g | Protein: 17 g | SmartPoints: 6 |

Sodium: If you use "no salt" added items for tomato sauce, stewed tomatoes & chicken/beef broth, it's 143mg sodium per serving.

INGREDIENTS

1 pound extra lean ground beef (could also use ground bison or moose)
1 medium onion, chopped
1 (14.5 oz) can stewed tomatoes
1 14oz can low sodium (or no salt added) tomato sauce
1 Tbsp minced garlic
1 Tbsp worchestershire sauce
1 cup low sodium chicken broth or beef broth
1 tsp black pepper
1/2 tsp hot chili flakes
1/2 head cabbage, chopped

DIRECTIONS

In a medium pot, brown beef & onions. Place everything in slow cooker (except meat mixture and cabbage) and mix well. Add beef mixture, then cabbage. Cook on LOW for 5-6 hours.

Veggie Shepherd's Pie cooked with creamy mashed cauliflower instead of potatoes (Be sure to save enough for tomorrow's lunch!)

Yields: 6 servings | Serving Size: 1 cup | Calories: 189 | Total Fat: 5 g | Saturated Fat: 2 g | Trans Fat: 0 g | Cholesterol: 6 mg | Sodium: 473mg | Carbohydrates: 23 g | Dietary Fiber: 7g | Sugars: 8 g | Protein: 19 g | SmartPoints: 5 |

INGREDIENTS

1 head of cauliflower, chopped

1/2 cup low-fat Greek yogurt

1 tablespoon pure butter

1 tablespoon olive oil

1 (12 ounce package) veggie soy crumbles (such as those from MorningStar Farms or Boca)

1/3 cup ketchup (recipe for Homemade Ketchup)

1 medium onion, diced

1 1/2 cup frozen peas and carrots

1 cup vegetable broth, low-sodium

1 tablespoon cornstarch

Sea salt and fresh ground black pepper, to taste

DIRECTIONS

Preheat oven to 400 degrees.

Lay the cauliflower on a parchment lined baking sheet. Spray lightly with cooking spray. Roast for 15-20 minutes until cauliflower is tender, but not mushy.Transfer cauliflower to the bowl of a food processor and add the yogurt and butter. Season with salt and pepper, and process until smooth and creamy.

Heat a skillet over medium high heat and add the olive oil. Add the veggie crumbles and cook until browned. Add the onion, carrots, and peas and stir until well combined. Combine the veggie broth with the cornstarch and stir until dissolved. Add this and the ketchup to the veggie mixture and stir.

Spread the vegetable mixture in a 8x8 casserole dish or divide into individual ramekins. Top with the pureed cauliflower and spread it on top.

Bake for 25 minutes until heated throughout. To brown the top, turn the broiler on high and broil until the top is browned to your liking. Alternatively, if you have a kitchen torch, you can use that to brown the top. Serve hot.

Snack/Dessert: Half cup mixed nuts

Slow Cooker Zucchini Ziti

Yields: 10 Servings | Serving Size: 3/4 Cup | Calories: 272 | Total Fat: 7 g | Saturated Fat: 3 g | Trans Fat: 0 | Cholesterol: 21 mg | Sodium: 376 mg | Carbohydrates: 38 g | Sugars: 7 g | Dietary Fiber: 5 g | Protein: 15 g | SmartPoints: 8 |

INGREDIENTS

1 (25 oz.) jar marinara (no sugar added)
3 cups (uncooked) whole grain ziti shells, optional penne
2 cups fat-free cottage cheese
2 cups mozzarella cheese, shredded
1 large zucchini (1/4" slices)
1/4 teaspoon black pepper
kosher or sea salt to taste
1/2 cup finely grated Parmesan cheese

DIRECTIONS

In a medium bowl combine the cottage cheese, mozzarella, and spices. Add one cup marinara to bottom of the slow cooker. Combine (uncooked) pasta shells with remaining marinara. Layer pasta coated marinara, zucchini, and cheese mixture until all ingredients have been used. Cheese should be the last ingredient added.

Cover and cook on low for two hours, or until pasta is al dente. Recommend using a 5 to 7 quart slow cooker.

Herby, Juicy Watermelon, Tomato and Feta Salad

Yields: 6 servings | Serving size: 1 cup| Calories: 162 | Total Fat: 10.4 gm | Saturated Fats: 4.5 gm | Trans Fats: 0.0 gm | Cholesterol: 22 mg | Sodium: 294 mg | Carbohydrates: 13.8 gm | Dietary fiber: 3.0 gm | Sugars: 9.7 gm | Protein: 5.2 gm| SmartPoints: 7

INGREDIENTS

1/2 large watermelon, balled (with a melon baller) or cubed (bite-size)
1 package feta cheese, cut into bite-size cubes
1 pint cherry tomatoes, halved (or 2 to 3 regular tomatoes, cut into bite size pieces)
2 red onions, cut in half and chopped into thin slices (for thin half slices)
3 tablespoons chopped fresh oregano
1/2 cup torn mint leaves
2 tablespoons red wine vinegar
2 tablespoons olive oil

DIRECTIONS

Put all of the salad ingredients into a large bowl as you are chopping, except for the olive oil and vinegar.

In a small bowl or a measuring cup, whisk together the olive oil and vinegar and pour into the salad and toss all of the ingredients together.

Chicken Noodle Soup cooked without noodles (Be sure to save enough for tomorrow's lunch!)

Yields: 8-10 servings | Serving Size: 1 cup |Calories: 174 | Total Fat: 3.6 g | Saturated Fat: 1.0 g | Trans Fat: 0 g | Cholesterol: 47 mg | Sodium: 78 mg | Carbohydrates: 16.7 g | Dietary Fiber: 2.4 g | Sugars: 1.2 g | Protein: 18.3 g | SmartPoints: 4

INGREDIENTS

1 tablespoon olive oil

2 medium carrots, chopped

3 medium celery stalks, trimmed and diced

1 medium white onion, diced

4 cups high quality (organic, low sodium) or homemade chicken stock

1 teaspoon black pepper

1 teaspoon garlic powder (or 2 cloves crushed)

1 teaspoon dill weed

1 rotisserie chicken

1 cup whole wheat egg noodles

3 tablespoons fresh parsley, minced

DIRECTIONS

In a pot that is able to hold at least 3 quarts, heat the olive oil over medium high heat. Add the mirepoix and saute for about 4 minutes, until the onion has softened.

While the vegetables are in the pot, disassemble the chicken: Remove the skin from the entire bird, save half and throw the other half away. Pull as much meat off of the bones that you can, set aside. Throw away all of the bones and large pieces of fat.

After the onion has softened, add the chicken stock, black pepper, garlic and dill weed. Bring back to a simmer over medium heat and simmer for 5-6 minutes.

Add in the reserved chicken skin, 1 cup of chicken meat and the noodles. Simmer for about 10 minutes until a light foam forms. Skim this foam with a spoon. Remove and discard the skin once the 10 minutes are up.

Taste now and determine if you need to add any salt or additional pepper. The rotisserie chicken should impart some salt, so you may not want to add any. I added 3 pinches to mine. Stir in the minced parsley. Serve hot with crackers.

*To keep gluten free: replace pasta with rice, quinoa or other grain free additive of your choice.

*To keep low carb, skip the noodles. It's still delish!

Pork Tenderloin with Peach Salsa and Peppery Slaw

Yields: 4 servings | Serving Size: 2 slices pork, 2 Tbsp salsa, and 1/2 cup slaw |Calories: 330 | Total Fat: 16.7 g | Saturated Fat: 3.2 g | Trans Fat: 0 g | Cholesterol: 83 mg | Sodium: 533 mg | Carbohydrates: 13.9 g | Dietary Fiber: 3.3 g | Sugars: 8.9 g | Protein: 31.5 g |SmartPoints: 9

INGREDIENTS

1 pound pork tenderloin, trimmed
2 tablespoons chopped fresh parsley, divided
1 tablespoon lemon zest
1 tablespoon minced garlic, divided
1 ½ teaspoons olive oil, divided
¾ teaspoon kosher salt, divided
¾ teaspoon black pepper, divided
1½ cups chopped fresh peaches
¼ cup chopped red onion
2 tablespoons lemon juice
1 tablespoon chopped fresh jalapeno
2 cups angel hair slaw
1 cup shredded carrots
⅓ cup cider vinegar
3 tablespoons extra virgin olive oil
1 teaspoon red pepper flakes
¼ teaspoon ground red pepper
Salt and pepper to taste

DIRECTIONS

Preheat grill to medium-high heat. Combine 1 tablespoon parsley, lemon zest, 2 teaspoons garlic, 1 teaspoon oil, ½ teaspoon salt, and ½ teaspoon pepper in a small bowl. Rub mixture evenly over pork. Let stand 30 minutes at room temperature. Grill pork 20-22 minutes or until desired degree of doneness. Remove from grill and let stand 15 minutes before slicing.

To prepare salsa, combine peaches, red onion, lemon juice, and jalapeno in a bowl. Stir in remaining 1 tablespoon parsley, 1 teaspoon garlic, ½ teaspoon oil and remaining ¼ teaspoon each salt and pepper.

Combine slaw and carrots in a bowl. In a separate bowl, combine vinegar, extra virgin olive oil, red pepper flakes, ground red pepper, and salt and pepper to taste. Pour vinegar mixture over cabbage mixture and toss to combine; let stand 30 minutes.

Serve peach salsa over pork and slaw alongside. Yields 4 servings.

Citrus and Spinach Salad with Creamy Lemon Dressing

Yields: 10 servings | Serving Size: 1 cup salad and 1-1/2 tablespoons dressing | Calories: 318 | Total Fat: 23 g | Saturated Fat: 3 g | Trans Fat: 0 g | Cholesterol: 1 mg | Sodium: 113 mg | Carbohydrates: 26 g | Dietary Fiber: 4 g | Sugars: 14 g | Protein: 7 g | SmartPoints: 12

INGREDIENTS

3 to 4 large beets
1 bulb fennel
2 oranges (navel or blood oranges)
2 pink grapefruits
2 packages baby arugula, mesclun (sometimes called spring greens mix), or baby spinach
2 radishes, thinly sliced

1 small red onion, thinly sliced
2 cups shelled, unsalted, untoasted pistachios
3 tablespoons honey
1/3 cup fresh lemon juice (juice from about 4 lemons)
2 teaspoons lemon zest
1 clove garlic, minced
1 teaspoon Dijon mustard
1/4 teaspoon salt
Freshly ground black pepper, to taste
1/2 cup extra virgin olive oil
1/2 cup nonfat or lowfat Greek yogurt

DIRECTIONS

Preheat oven to 400 degrees. Scrub beets clean and wrap each tightly with foil. Do not peel the beets. Bake beets for about an hour until they are tender when pierced with a fork. Remove from the oven and allow to rest until they are cool enough to handle. Carefully removed the foil and peel the beets with a vegetable peeler. Slice the beets into even rounds.

To make citrus segments, first peel the citrus by placing it on a flat cutting board and cutting around it with a knife to remove both the peel and the white pith. Holding each piece of citrus at a bowl, one at a time, cut between each membrane of the fruit until a segment pops out. Strain the fruit and remove any seeds.

Alternatively, peel the citrus by hand and serve the segments in the salad with the skin on.

Using a sharp knife, slice the fennel horizontally as thinly as possible. Slice radishes across, very thinly as well.

Toast the pistachios by placing them in a saute pan or skillet over medium heat. It may be necessary to work in 2 batches so as not to crowd the pan. Stir constantly. Nuts should become fragrant and slightly golden brown after about 3 to 4 minutes. Pour the honey onto the nuts, stirring. Once the nuts are coated, take the skillet off the heat. Remove the nuts from the pan and place them flat on wax paper. Sprinkle with salt. Allow to cool for about 20 to 30 minutes to harden.

In a large bowl, combine the arugula, fennel, radishes, onion, and citrus.

Combine the lemon juice, lemon zest, garlic, dijon mustard, and salt and pepper in a bowl. Drizzle the olive oil in a gradual stream, whisking the whole time. Next, whisk in the Greek yogurt.

Add the beets to the top or along the sides of the salad (the rich color bleeds into the salad). Sprinkle the candied pistachios on top of the salad. Serve the dressing on the side, or drizzle over just before serving.

Slow Cooker Black Bean and Chicken served in a low-carb tortilla (Be sure to save enough for tomorrow's lunch!)

Yields: 9 Servings | Serving Size: 1/2 cup | Calories: 276 | Total Fat: 8 g | Saturated Fats: 2 g | Trans Fats: 0 g | Cholesterol: 32 mg | Sodium: 827 mg | Carbohydrates: 33 g | Dietary Fiber: 5 g | Sugars: 4 g | Protein: 18 g | SmartPoints: 6 |

INGREDIENTS

4 chicken breast fillets (1 pound), skinless, boneless
1 (15 ounce) can black beans, drained
2 cups salsa of your choice
8 tortillas, whole wheat or low carb

DIRECTIONS

Add all ingredients to the slow cooker, except tortillas. Cook on low for 4-6 hours. Shred it with a fork. Serve in a low carb tortilla, by itself or over a salad. Kids will love this one.

Paleo Friendly Meaty Veggie Roll-ups

Yields: 12 roll-ups | Serving Size: 4-6 roll ups |Calories: 71 | Total Fat: 2.0 g | Saturated Fat: 0.6 g | Trans Fat: 0 g | Cholesterol: 29 mg | Sodium: 27 mg | Carbohydrates: 1.2 g | Dietary Fiber: 0 g | Sugars: 0.8 g | Protein: 11.3g | SmartPoints: 1

INGREDIENTS

12 thick slices unprocessed deli meat, we recommend Boar's Head Brand
1 cup sliced vegetables
12 chives, optional

DIRECTIONS

Place desired amount of vegetables on a piece of deli meat. Roll tightly, and if desired, use a chive to tie. Pack in a zip-top plastic bag or airtight container.

Favorite Flavor Combinations:

Roast beef with red bell pepper strips, carrot sticks, and cucumber slices with mustard for dipping.

Chicken with apple slices, red cabbage, and pickle strips with Dijon mustard for dipping.

Turkey with crumbled bacon and sliced avocado with salsa for dipping.

Slow Cooke Lower Carb Cabbage Roll Stew (Be sure to save enough for tomorrow's lunch!)

Yields: 6 Servings | Serving Size: 1 1/3 Cup | Calories: 242 | Fat: 13 g | Carbohydrates: 14 g | Fiber: 3 g | Sugars: 6 g | Protein: 17 g | SmartPoints: 6 |

Sodium: If you use "no salt" added items for tomato sauce, stewed tomatoes & chicken/beef broth, it's 143mg sodium per serving.

INGREDIENTS

1 pound extra lean ground beef (could also use ground bison or moose)
1 medium onion, chopped
1 (14.5 oz) can stewed tomatoes
1 14oz can low sodium (or no salt added) tomato sauce
1 Tbsp minced garlic
1 Tbsp worchestershire sauce
1 cup low sodium chicken broth or beef broth
1 tsp black pepper
1/2 tsp hot chili flakes
1/2 head cabbage, chopped

DIRECTIONS

In a medium pot, brown beef & onions. Place everything in slow cooker (except meat mixture and cabbage) and mix well. Add beef mixture, then cabbage. Cook on LOW for 5-6 hours.

Veggie Shepherd's Pie cooked with creamy mashed cauliflower

Yields: 6 servings | Serving Size: 1 cup | Calories: 189 | Total Fat: 5 g | Saturated Fat: 2 g | Trans Fat: 0 g | Cholesterol: 6 mg | Sodium: 473mg | Carbohydrates: 23 g | Dietary Fiber: 7g | Sugars: 8 g | Protein: 19 g | SmartPoints: 5 |

INGREDIENTS

1 head of cauliflower, chopped
1/2 cup low-fat Greek yogurt
1 tablespoon pure butter
1 tablespoon olive oil
1 (12 ounce package) veggie soy crumbles (such as those from MorningStar Farms or Boca)
1/3 cup ketchup (recipe for Homemade Ketchup)
1 medium onion, diced
1 1/2 cup frozen peas and carrots
1 cup vegetable broth, low-sodium
1 tablespoon cornstarch
Sea salt and fresh ground black pepper, to taste

DIRECTIONS

Preheat oven to 400 degrees.

Lay the cauliflower on a parchment lined baking sheet. Spray lightly with cooking spray. Roast for 15-20 minutes until cauliflower is tender, but not mushy.Transfer cauliflower to the bowl of a food processor and add the yogurt and butter. Season with salt and pepper, and process until smooth and creamy.

Heat a skillet over medium high heat and add the olive oil. Add the veggie crumbles and cook until browned. Add the onion, carrots, and peas and stir until well combined. Combine the veggie broth with the cornstarch and stir until dissolved. Add this and the ketchup to the veggie mixture and stir.

Spread the vegetable mixture in a 8x8 casserole dish or divide into individual ramekins. Top with the pureed cauliflower and spread it on top.

Bake for 25 minutes until heated throughout. To brown the top, turn the broiler on high and broil until the top is browned to your liking. Alternatively, if you have a kitchen torch, you can use that to brown the top. Serve hot.

Snack/Dessert: Half cup mixed nuts

Slow Cooker Zucchini Ziti

Yields: 10 Servings | Serving Size: 3/4 Cup | Calories: 272 | Total Fat: 7 g | Saturated Fat: 3 g | Trans Fat: 0 | Cholesterol: 21 mg | Sodium: 376 mg | Carbohydrates: 38 g | Sugars: 7 g | Dietary Fiber: 5 g | Protein: 15 g | SmartPoints: 8 |

INGREDIENTS

1 (25 oz.) jar marinara (no sugar added)
3 cups (uncooked) whole grain ziti shells, optional penne
2 cups fat-free cottage cheese
2 cups mozzarella cheese, shredded
1 large zucchini (1/4" slices)
1/4 teaspoon black pepper
kosher or sea salt to taste
1/2 cup finely grated Parmesan cheese

DIRECTIONS

In a medium bowl combine the cottage cheese, mozzarella, and spices. Add one cup marinara to bottom of the slow cooker. Combine (uncooked) pasta shells with remaining marinara. Layer pasta coated marinara, zucchini, and cheese mixture until all ingredients have been used. Cheese should be the last ingredient added.

Cover and cook on low for two hours, or until pasta is al dente. Recommend using a 5 to 7 quart slow cooker.

Strawberry Banana Smoothie

Servings: 2 | Serving Size: 1/2 of the entire recipe | Calories: 250 | Total Fat: 5 g | Saturated Fats: 0 g | Trans Fats: 0 g | Cholesterol: 13 mg | Sodium: 28 mg | Carbohydrates: 41 g | Dietary fiber: 5.5 g | Sugars: 21 g | Protein: 13 g | SmartPoints: 9 |

INGREDIENTS

1 large frozen banana (slice into 1? pieces before freezing)
6 large frozen strawberries (unsweetened)
1/2 slice fresh ginger root (optional)
1 cup skim milk (almond or milk alternative**)
½ cup Greek Yogurt, plain fat free
1/4 cup wheat germ

DIRECTIONS

Place all the ingredients in a blender and blend until creamy…just like a milkshake. Add a straw and enjoy!

Herby, Juicy Watermelon, Tomato and Feta Salad

Yields: 6 servings | Serving size: 1 cup| Calories: 162 | Total Fat: 10.4 gm | Saturated Fats: 4.5 gm | Trans Fats: 0.0 gm | Cholesterol: 22 mg | Sodium: 294 mg | Carbohydrates: 13.8 gm | Dietary fiber: 3.0 gm | Sugars: 9.7 gm | Protein: 5.2 gm| SmartPoints: 7

INGREDIENTS

1/2 large watermelon, balled (with a melon baller) or cubed (bite-size)
1 package feta cheese, cut into bite-size cubes
1 pint cherry tomatoes, halved (or 2 to 3 regular tomatoes, cut into bite size pieces)
2 red onions, cut in half and chopped into thin slices (for thin half slices)

3 tablespoons chopped fresh oregano
1/2 cup torn mint leaves
2 tablespoons red wine vinegar
2 tablespoons olive oil

DIRECTIONS

Put all of the salad ingredients into a large bowl as you are chopping, except for the olive oil and vinegar.

In a small bowl or a measuring cup, whisk together the olive oil and vinegar and pour into the salad and toss all of the ingredients together.

Chicken Noodle Soup cooked without noodles

Yields: 8-10 servings | Serving Size: 1 cup |Calories: 174 | Total Fat: 3.6 g | Saturated Fat: 1.0 g | Trans Fat: 0 g | Cholesterol: 47 mg | Sodium: 78 mg | Carbohydrates: 16.7 g | Dietary Fiber: 2.4 g | Sugars: 1.2 g | Protein: 18.3 g | SmartPoints: 4

INGREDIENTS

1 tablespoon olive oil
2 medium carrots, chopped
3 medium celery stalks, trimmed and diced
1 medium white onion, diced
4 cups high quality (organic, low sodium) or homemade chicken stock
1 teaspoon black pepper
1 teaspoon garlic powder (or 2 cloves crushed)
1 teaspoon dill weed
1 rotisserie chicken
1 cup whole wheat egg noodles
3 tablespoons fresh parsley, minced

DIRECTIONS

In a pot that is able to hold at least 3 *q*uarts, heat the olive oil over medium high heat. Add the mirepoix and saute for about 4 minutes, until the onion has softened.

While the vegetables are in the pot, disassemble the chicken: Remove the skin from the entire bird, save half and throw the other half away. Pull as much meat off of the bones that you can, set aside. Throw away all of the bones and large pieces of fat.

After the onion has softened, add the chicken stock, black pepper, garlic and dill weed. Bring back to a simmer over medium heat and simmer for 5-6 minutes.

Add in the reserved chicken skin, 1 cup of chicken meat and the noodles. Simmer for about 10 minutes until a light foam forms. Skim this foam with a spoon. Remove and discard the skin once the 10 minutes are up.

Taste now and determine if you need to add any salt or additional pepper. The rotisserie chicken should impart some salt, so you may not want to add any. I added 3 pinches to mine. Stir in the minced parsley. Serve hot with crackers.

*To keep gluten free: replace pasta with rice, quinoa or other grain free additive of your choice.

*To keep low carb, skip the noodles. It's still delish!

Pork Tenderloin with Peach Salsa and Peppery Slaw

Yields: 4 servings | Serving Size: 2 slices pork, 2 Tbsp salsa, and 1/2 cup slaw |Calories: 330 | Total Fat: 16.7 g | Saturated Fat: 3.2 g | Trans Fat: 0 g | Cholesterol: 83 mg | Sodium: 533 mg | Carbohydrates: 13.9 g | Dietary Fiber: 3.3 g | Sugars: 8.9 g | Protein: 31.5 g |SmartPoints: 9

INGREDIENTS

1 pound pork tenderloin, trimmed

2 tablespoons chopped fresh parsley, divided

1 tablespoon lemon zest

1 tablespoon minced garlic, divided

1 ½ teaspoons olive oil, divided

¾ teaspoon kosher salt, divided

¾ teaspoon black pepper, divided

1½ cups chopped fresh peaches

¼ cup chopped red onion

2 tablespoons lemon juice

1 tablespoon chopped fresh jalapeno

2 cups angel hair slaw

1 cup shredded carrots

⅓ cup cider vinegar

3 tablespoons extra virgin olive oil

1 teaspoon red pepper flakes

¼ teaspoon ground red pepper

Salt and pepper to taste

DIRECTIONS

Preheat grill to medium-high heat. Combine 1 tablespoon parsley, lemon zest, 2 teaspoons garlic, 1 teaspoon oil, ½ teaspoon salt, and ½ teaspoon pepper in a small bowl. Rub mixture evenly over pork. Let stand 30 minutes at room temperature. Grill pork 20-22 minutes or until desired degree of doneness. Remove from grill and let stand 15 minutes before slicing.

To prepare salsa, combine peaches, red onion, lemon juice, and jalapeno in a bowl. Stir in remaining 1 tablespoon parsley, 1 teaspoon garlic, ½ teaspoon oil and remaining ¼ teaspoon each salt and pepper.

Combine slaw and carrots in a bowl. In a separate bowl, combine vinegar, extra virgin olive oil, red pepper flakes, ground red pepper, and salt and pepper to taste. Pour vinegar mixture over cabbage mixture and toss to combine; let stand 30 minutes.

Serve peach salsa over pork and slaw alongside. Yields 4 servings.

Citrus and Spinach Salad with Creamy Lemon Dressing

Yields: 10 servings | Serving Size: 1 cup salad and 1-1/2 tablespoons dressing | Calories: 318 | Total Fat: 23 g | Saturated Fat: 3 g | Trans Fat: 0 g | Cholesterol: 1 mg | Sodium: 113 mg | Carbohydrates: 26 g | Dietary Fiber: 4 g | Sugars: 14 g | Protein: 7 g | SmartPoints: 12

INGREDIENTS

3 to 4 large beets
1 bulb fennel
2 oranges (navel or blood oranges)
2 pink grapefruits
2 packages baby arugula, mesclun (sometimes called spring greens mix), or baby spinach
2 radishes, thinly sliced
1 small red onion, thinly sliced
2 cups shelled, unsalted, untoasted pistachios
3 tablespoons honey
1/3 cup fresh lemon juice (juice from about 4 lemons)
2 teaspoons lemon zest
1 clove garlic, minced
1 teaspoon Dijon mustard
1/4 teaspoon salt
Freshly ground black pepper, to taste
1/2 cup extra virgin olive oil
1/2 cup nonfat or lowfat Greek yogurt

DIRECTIONS

Preheat oven to 400 degrees. Scrub beets clean and wrap each tightly with foil. Do not peel the beets. Bake beets for about an hour until they are tender when pierced with a fork. Remove from the oven and allow to rest until they are cool enough to handle. Carefully removed the foil and peel the beets with a vegetable peeler. Slice the beets into even rounds.

To make citrus segments, first peel the citrus by placing it on a flat cutting board and cutting around it with a knife to remove both the peel and the white pith. Holding each piece of citrus at a bowl, one at a time, cut between each membrane of the fruit until a segment pops out. Strain the fruit and remove any seeds.

Alternatively, peel the citrus by hand and serve the segments in the salad with the skin on.

Using a sharp knife, slice the fennel horizontally as thinly as possible. Slice radishes across, very thinly as well.

Toast the pistachios by placing them in a saute pan or skillet over medium heat. It may be necessary to work in 2 batches so as not to crowd the pan. Stir constantly. Nuts should become fragrant and slightly golden brown after about 3 to 4 minutes. Pour the honey onto the nuts, stirring. Once the nuts are coated, take the skillet off the heat. Remove the nuts from the pan and place them flat on wax paper. Sprinkle with salt. Allow to cool for about 20 to 30 minutes to harden.

In a large bowl, combine the arugula, fennel, radishes, onion, and citrus.

Combine the lemon juice, lemon zest, garlic, dijon mustard, and salt and pepper in a bowl. Drizzle the olive oil in a gradual stream, whisking the whole time. Next, whisk in the Greek yogurt.

Add the beets to the top or along the sides of the salad (the rich color bleeds into the salad). Sprinkle the candied pistachios on top of the salad. Serve the dressing on the side, or drizzle over just before serving.

Slow Cooker Black Bean and Chicken served in a low-carb tortilla (Be sure to save enough for tomorrow's lunch!)

Yields: 9 Servings | Serving Size: 1/2 cup | Calories: 276 | Total Fat: 8 g | Saturated Fats: 2 g | Trans Fats: 0 g | Cholesterol: 32 mg | Sodium: 827 mg | Carbohydrates: 33 g | Dietary Fiber: 5 g | Sugars: 4 g | Protein: 18 g | SmartPoints: 6 |

INGREDIENTS

4 chicken breast fillets (1 pound), skinless, boneless
1 (15 ounce) can black beans, drained
2 cups salsa of your choice
8 tortillas, whole wheat or low carb

DIRECTIONS

Add all ingredients to the slow cooker, except tortillas. Cook on low for 4-6 hours. Shred it with a fork. Serve in a low carb tortilla, by itself or over a salad. Kids will love this one.

Slow Cooker Black Bean and Chicken served in a low-carb tortilla (Left over from last night's dinner)

Yields: 10 | Serving size: 1 cup | Calories: 192 | Total Fat: 3 g | Saturated Fats: 1 g | Trans Fats: 0 g | Cholesterol: 37 mg | Sodium: 202 mg | Carbohydrates: 21 g | Dietary fiber: 6 g | Sugars: 2 g | Protein: 20 g | SmartPoints: 4 |

INGREDIENTS

1/2 cup diced onion

1 clove garlic, minced

1 (15 oz.) can black beans, rinsed and drained

1 (15 oz.) can kidney beans|, rinsed and drained

1 (4.5 oz.) can diced green chili peppers

1 (14.5 oz.) can diced tomatoes

2 1/2 cups chicken broth, low sodium, fat-free (use more broth for a thinner soup)

1 cup frozen or fresh corn

Juice from 1 lime

1 tablespoon chili powder

1 teaspoon cumin

1/2 teaspoon cayenne pepper (more or less to taste)

1/2 teaspoon black pepper

Kosher or sea salt to taste

1/2 cup freshly chopped cilantro

2 chicken breasts fillets, skinless, cut into 1-2" cubes (no need to pre-cook)

DIRECTIONS

Add all ingredients to the slow cooker, stir to combine. Cover and cook on low 6-8 hours.

Chapter 9: Snacks & Desserts:

Zucchini Hummus with fresh veggies

Yields: 8-10 servings | Serving Size: 2 Tbsp |Calories: 140 | Total Fat:13.4 g | Saturated Fat: 1.9 g | Trans Fat: 0 g | Cholesterol: 0 mg | Sodium: 20 mg | Carbohydrates: 4.5 g | Dietary Fiber: 1.6 g | Sugars: 0.6 g | Protein: 2.7 g | SmartPoints: 5

INGREDIENTS

2 medium zucchini, peeled and chopped
½ cup tahini
⅓ cup lemon juice
⅓ cup olive oil
3 garlic cloves
1½ teaspoons cumin
Sea Salt & pepper to taste

DIRECTIONS

Combine all ingredients in the base of a food processor, and process until smooth. Serve with crisp raw veggies, such as carrots, celery sticks, broccoli, cherry tomatoes, or cucumber slices, for dipping.

Clean-Eating Caramel Apples

Yields: 10 servings | Serving Size: 1 candied apple | Calories: 161 | Total Fat: 4 g | Saturated Fat: 3 g | Trans Fat: 0 g | Cholesterol: 0 mg |

Sodium: 73 mg | Carbohydrates: 32 g | Dietary Fiber: 4 g | Sugars: 13 g | Protein: 2 g | SmartPoints: 7

INGREDIENTS

10 small-variety apples such as lady apples or 6 large apples such as Granny Smith or McIntosh
1/3 cup coconut milk
1 cup brown rice syrup
2 teaspoons real vanilla extract
1 tablespoon coconut oil, or good quality unsalted butter
1/4 teaspoon salt

DIRECTIONS

Wash and dry each apple. Insert bamboo skewers, or wooden sticks into the bottom end of each apple. Pull the stem from the top of each apple to remove.

Whisk the coconut milk, coconut oil and brown rice syrup in a medium saucepan over medium--low heat. Allow to cook for 10 minutes. The sauce should bubble. Whisk in salt, vanilla, and coconut oil or butter.

Remove the caramel sauce from the heat. The caramel will thicken upon standing. Roll the apples in the caramel and use a spoon to pour on, and the back of the spoon to spread.

Set each skewered caramel apple onto wax paper lined baking sheet. Allow to set in the fridge for an hour to harden. Place lined or grouped on a plate to serve.

Angel Eggs (Classic Deviled Eggs Recipe)
INGREDIENTS
- 2 large eggs

- ¼ cup reduced fat mayonnaise
- ¼ tablespoon Dijon mustard
- 1 sprigs fresh dill + extra for garnish
- ½ teaspoons diced shallots
- ½ teaspoon hot smoked paprika
- ½ teaspoon salt
- ¼ teaspoon pepper
- ½ tablespoons capers

DIRECTIONS

Place 2 eggs in a pot. Fill the pot with cold water until it covers the eggs by about an inch. Bring the water to a boil; then reduce to a low simmer for 15 minutes. Remove the pot from the stove and place it in the sink. Run cold water into the pot for several minutes until the pot is full of cold water. Remove the eggs. Roll each egg to crack the shell and gently peel.

With a sharp knife, cut each egg in half length-wise. Remove the yolks and place them in the food processor. Add the mayo, mustard, dill, shallots, paprika, salt and pepper to the egg yolks. Puree until extremely smooth.

Using a pastry bag and tip, or a zip-bag with one corner snipped off, pipe the yolk mixture into the hole of each egg. Sprinkle a few capers and extra chopped dill on each egg. Cover and refrigerate until ready to eat.

Shrimp and Scallop Scampi with Linguine
INGREDIENTS
- Kosher salt
- 1 pound linguine
- 12 jumbo shrimp, peeled and deveined
- 12 large sea scallops, tough foot muscles removed
- Freshly ground pepper

- 3 1/2 tablespoons unsalted butter
- 2 cloves garlic, minced
- 2 tablespoons fresh lemon juice, plus lemon wedges for garnish
- 1/2 cup dry white wine
- 1/4 cup torn fresh basil
- 2 tablespoons chopped fresh parsley

DIRECTIONS

Bring a large pot of salted water to a boil. Add the linguine and cook as the label directs.

Meanwhile, heat a large skillet over medium-high heat. Pat the shrimp and scallops dry, then season with salt and pepper. Add 1 1/2 tablespoons butter to the pan and cook the shrimp until golden on one side, about 3 minutes. Turn the shrimp and add half of the garlic; cook until the garlic is fragrant but the shrimp are still translucent, 1 to 2 more minutes. Transfer the shrimp to a plate.

Add the scallops to the skillet and cook until golden on one side, about 3 minutes. Turn the scallops, add the remaining garlic and cook 1 to 2 more minutes. Add the lemon juice and wine and bring to a boil, scraping up any browned bits with a wooden spoon. Cook until the sauce is reduced by half, about 3 minutes. Return the shrimp to the pan, then add the basil and the remaining 2 tablespoons butter; season with salt and pepper.

Drain the pasta and transfer to a large serving bowl. Toss with the shrimp, scallops and sauce; garnish with parsley and lemon

Oven Baked Beet Chips Recipe
INGREDIENTS
- 3 beets (red, golden, or mixed)
- ¼ cup olive oil
- ¼ teaspoon celery salt (or sea salt)

DIRECTIONS

Preheat the oven to 300 degrees F, and line several baking sheets with parchment paper. Scrub the beets well with a veggie brush and cut off the tops.

Use a mandolin slicer to slice the beets paper-thin (1/16 inch.) When the beet slices are this thin, there is no need to peel them first. Hold the root end while dragging the beets across the mandolin and watch your finger tips closely.

Place the beet slices in a large bowl and pour the oil and salt over the top. Toss well. (If using red and golden beets, place in separate bowls and divide the oil and salt evenly.) Ready for the secret step? Now let the beets sit in the oil and salt until they release there natural juices, about 15-20 minutes. This is what allows them to retain a better shape and color.

Toss the beets again, then drain off the liquid. Lay the slices out in a single layer on the prepared baking sheets. Bake for 45-60 minutes until crisp, but not brown. Test after 45 minutes and only bake longer if necessary. Remove the beet chips from the oven and cool completely before storing in an air-tight container.

Peanut Butter Banana Quesadillas
INGREDIENTS
- 1 8-inch whole wheat tortilla
- 2 Tbsp natural peanut butter
- ½ medium banana
- 1 Tbsp semi-sweet chocolate chips

DIRECTIONS

Spread the peanut butter over the surface of the tortilla.

Slice the banana very thinly and then arrange the slices over half of the tortilla. Sprinkle the chocolate chips over the banana slices and then fold the tortilla in half.

Cook the quesadilla in a skillet over medium-low heat until golden brown and crispy on both sides.

Truck-Stop Buttermilk Pancakes

INGREDIENTS
- 5 eggs
- 1 1/2 cups milk
- 6 tablespoons butter, melted
- 5 cups buttermilk
- 5 cups all-purpose flour
- 5 teaspoons baking powder
- 5 teaspoons baking soda
- 1 pinch salt (optional)
- 5 tablespoons sugar

DIRECTIONS

In a large bowl, whisk together the eggs, milk, butter and buttermilk. Combine the flour, baking powder, baking soda and sugar; stir into the wet ingredients just until blended. Adjust the thickness of the batter to your liking by adding more flour or buttermilk if necessary.

Heat a large skillet over medium heat, and coat with cooking spray. Pour 1/4 cupfuls of batter onto the skillet, and cook until bubbles appear on the surface. Flip with a spatula, and cook until browned on the other side. Continue with remaining batter.

Slow Cooker Beets with Creamy Goat Cheese Sauce

Yield: 4 beets | Serving Size: 1 beet |Calories: 203 | Total Fat: 13.8 g | Saturated Fat: 7.5 g | Trans Fat: 0 g | Cholesterol: 30 mg | Sodium:175

mg | Carbohydrates: 10.8 g | Dietary Fiber: 2.1 g | Sugars: 8.6 g | Protein: 10.4 g | SmartPoints: 8

INGREDIENTS

4 beets
1 tbsp olive oil
Salt, to taste
Pepper, to taste
Goat Cheese Spread
4 oz. soft goat cheese
1 tbsp olive oil
1 tsp each fresh basil and thyme

DIRECTIONS

Begin by scrubbing the exterior of the beet to remove any dirt from the skin. Remove tops from the beets.

Make 4, 6" x 6" squares of aluminum foil. Place a beet in the center of each square.

Drizzle beets with olive oil and just a sprinkling of salt and pepper. Wrap the foil around the beet until it is completely enclosed.

Place beets in your slow cooker and cook on high for 4 hours.

For the Goat Cheese Sauce, combine the cheese olive oil, basil, and thyme in a blender. Blend until smooth. Refrigerate until ready to use.

When removing the packages from the slow cooker, carefully open the aluminum foil and allow any steam to escape (they will be very hot!!)

Once the beets are cool, remove the skins with a small knife – the skins should just fall off. Serve with goat cheese sauce and fresh basil. Enjoy!

Made in the USA
Columbia, SC
03 April 2019